A Practical Guide to Health from One
of the Country's Top Fitness Experts

AFFIRM
FITNESS

BODY • MIND • SPIRIT

50 tips to a fitter more whole+sum you !!

TEDDY BASS

& Amika Ryan

Cover and book design by Amika Ryan
Cover Image © 2016 by Michael Muller
Author photographs by Michael Muller and Orion Shrader

Chapter opening illustrations © by gorbach elena/ Benjavisa Ruangvaree/Andrey tiyk/ibreakstock at Shutterstock

Hey,

Welcome to this wonderful book brought to you by That Guy's House Publishing.

At That Guy's House we believe in real and raw wellness books that inspire the reader from a place of authenticity and honesty.

This book has been carefully crafted by both the author and publisher with the intention that it will bring you a glimmer of hope, a rush of inspiration and sensation of inner peace.

It is our hope that you thoroughly enjoy this book and pass it onto friends who may also be in need of a glimpse into their own magnificence.

Have a wonderful day.

Love,

Sean Patrick
That Guy.

Rachel, Together always working + Hoping to assist and support - support these tips + affirmations graceful you, the most of you, Rachel in the journey in the way, let this journey towards the your being towards whole + Sum you. fitter more !!

To my first impressions of love -
my mother and four sisters.
T.B.

To all the women in my life who turned out to be more
than just clients, but also dear friends.
A.R.

CONTENTS

ACKNOWLEDGMENTS

There are people that have been delivered into my life that have touched it, and gifted to me experiences that have brought me to this moment. I am beyond grateful for each and every one of them, and there are a great many of them! These people have supported me along this journey called life, and are the inspiration of the creation of this very special book. Each of them, giving a small part of themselves, has made this book a kaleidoscope of love, light, and wisdom. I wish to thank all of them for assisting me in my dream of helping others to reach their greatest potential and most vibrant health.

Helen Hughes and Ted Bass, my parents, for the decision to keep trying for a boy after having four girls. They finally got it right, and here I am. They have gifted me with so many life lessons and opportunities that I otherwise would not have received.

David, my life, my son, who has invited invaluable growth into my life. I'm grateful for him, beyond words, for the love and expansion he has given me.

Adrienne, my second mother, and her husband, Ricky, of 40 years, who have been parental figures, who helped raise me and support me through my life's endeavors.

Marsha, the nurse who followed in my mother's footsteps, saving the world, one child at a time. Her big, loving heart has taught me so much.

Christye, with her big heart and quiet soul, gave me such great insights about things that others could not.

Suzanna, my sister and friend, who shares with me a deep love of God. Her constituted desire to let go, and raise the vibration of the world to foster greater love and peace for all my sisters, for making me into the man and father I am today.

All of the children that I call "niece" and "nephew". Each has a special place in my ever-expanding heart.

Janet, my son's godmother, for the long-term friendship and modeling of a true, unconditionally loving parent. She is an important mentor in my life and has always supported me.

Christina, for being the longest training relationship I have in my life. She introduced me to the most transformational spiritual community, Agape International Spiritual Center, which has shaped my adult life and put me on the quest of growth and transformation. And she introduced me to many of my friends and clients over the years.

Cameron, the second-longest-term relationship of my life. She is a powerful woman, with a voice and desire to parallel my own journey of growth and inner transformation. She inspires me each day.

Lucy, no matter how near or far, your constant friendship is like a lifeline. She demonstrated progress and growth towards the ever expanding good in life. Her presence is more than valuable to me, it is necessary.

Michael Bernard Beckwith, minister and teacher, and Rickie Byars Beckwith, healer through song and choir director, both my teachers of truth and music. They have helped me to serve in many capacities over the last 20 years: to support others, find freedom through spiritual practices like prayer treatment, mediation, visioning, tithing and service.

Jessica and Bryan, for the summers they have spent with my son, and allowing him to experience a southern vacation.

Kathleen McNamara, my teacher, spiritual mentor, fellow practitioner and dearest friend. Almost all great things in my life have involved her in some way. Her loyalty and spiritual integrity are miraculous.

Stefania Magidson, my dearest angel. We have worked together for over 15 years, and she has never been afraid to disagree with me. She is my soldier on this journey of life and truth seeking. She is a mirror and confidant that makes my life just a little sweeter.

Soliel and Heather, my two sisters separated at birth. They are my soulmates who support me in all that I do. I am Grateful for the depth of love and support they have always provided me.

Karen, my Berlin friend, who has been a light and rock in life with a heart of gold.

Julie, my longest journey of deep friendship. We have experienced many ups and downs, but prayer and faith keep us united. She is the mother of my godson, Nicholas, who is one of the reasons I decided to become a father.

Kim, my fellow Agape Spiritual Therapist Practitioner. At first meeting, I knew she was a lifer. What we share is irreplaceable.

Candice, a true prayer partner and life-long friend. She has supported me in freeing myself from old patterns and behaviors. She is a true warrior of life.

Paul Reaney, a British soul who showed me the meaning of BFF. He has supported me in my career, failed relationships, and parenting mishaps. He is the one I can always count on, no matter what. My brother from another mother, Joan Reaney.

Sutton, my southern gal-pal. We may live in the west coast, but we are both southern born and raised.

Amika Ryan, a friend who knows the real me, and puts my voice into words on paper. Our long-time friendship has evolved into a deep spiritual bond that combines fitness, personal growth and vision. We will continue to accomplish our goals, together.

T.B.

INTRODUCTION

Fitness today is a vast multi-billion dollar industry that can be challenging for any individual to navigate. Amidst your busy work or home schedule (finding time to eat, shop, nurture relationships, etc.), it is difficult to find time to focus on all of the ever-changing advice of health professionals.

Increasingly, people are finding it daunting to keep up with their own health, and are disjointed physically, mentally, and spiritually. This leads to overeating, under-sleeping, reactiveness, conflict, unhappiness, exhaustion, and burn-out. If you are one of these people, you're in luck because I wrote this book for you!

In my own life, the road of least resistance has not been one that I often took. I found a strange sort of comfort and familiarity in my constant struggles. In addition, I allowed my fear of change and the unknown to take hold. This all worked together to stunt my personal growth, and hindered my exploration into blissful abundance of many years.

I desperately wanted to expand my awareness and allow prosperity into all areas of my life, but I didn't know where to start. That's why I wrote this book.

Whatever change you feel that you need in your life right now, this book will help to usher you into that new existence. Change isn't easy but with your own desire and by following the guidance in this book, you can shift away from old behaviors, gain insight into yourself, and live a more healthy, stress-free existence.

True health and vitality are difficult to achieve without a wholesome existence. A seamless integration of body, mind, and spirit that is aligned with your *truth* is the only way to combat the heath epidemic in our society today.

I recently turned fifty-something years old and I feel like my authentic life is just now beginning. I have spent the last two decades as a professional in the health and fitness industry, figuring out just the right recipe for a joyous and healthy life. On my journey of transformation and physical well-being I have acquired many tools that have helped me reach a wonderful place of peace as well. The journey is ongoing, not always easy, and always rewarding.

Affirmed Fitness gives you a clear roadmap of what you can do today to align you body, mind, and spirit for a vibrant existence. Learn to increase your energy, improve immunity, heighten your mood, decrease stress, attract what you desire, and prolong your life with a happier and healthier body, mind, and spirit. The tips contained in these pages are made actionable, with a *Take Action* exercise, and each tip has its own *Affirmotion*.

Yes, *Affirmotion*, that's not a type-o. Affirmotions™ are affirmations that put YOU in motion! The Affirmotions™ take your intention for growth one step further by truly activating the positive new behavior or desired change that you desire. Taking words and activating them as a living demonstration, deep into your consciousness, will catapult your subconscious into change.

Affirmed Fitness offers up a recipe of success, putting your body, mind, and spirit into action, with *Take Action* exercises that accompany each tip in this book. This gives you a tangible directive that you can implement into your day, each and every day, turning healthy living into a habit.

I invite you to make these tips your own by customizing the *Take Action* exercises and *Affirmotion* statements to make them resonate with your authentic self.

For those those of you who are approaching, or are in your fifties, check out the *Bonus Chapter*, because there are a few tips back there tailored specifically to you.

I used to be *the master of distraction*. Too often, I got sidetracked from my greater purpose and resisted healthy change. These tips helped me to reach for my highest potential in health and life. I got more clear about the changes I needed to make, and closer each day to fulfilling my highest good in this life with gratitude and grace. Today, my hearts desire is to uplift and motivate you to reach your highest potential, no matter what!

I'm grateful that you've decided to take this journey into your healthier life by picking up this book. I hope that this book inspires you to be the best version of yourself, eases your transition, and contributes to a more enlightened existence. I want you to feel energized, in control, happy, informed, and that you can do and have anything your heart desires. This is your chance to let go of the past and to live your life, big and bold. At the end of this book you will be able to dance like nobody is watching!

- Teddy Bass

Learn more at

Affirmotions.com

Teddybass.com

ABOUT THE AUTHORS

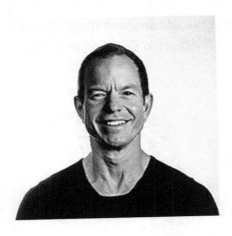

Teddy Bass is a certified member of the National Academy of Sports Medicine (NASM), and actively continues his studies at national fitness seminars focusing on pilates, nutrition, kinesiology, strength training, flexibility, and biomechanics. Teddy has been a spiritual therapist at Agape for over fifteen years. Teddy's life journey as a dancer and personal trainer for over twenty-three years has facilitated his life's work - to assist people in getting their vibrant, authentic lives back.

Teddy's training philosophy is a lifestyle, as opposed to a trend. He believes that setting goals creates an inner determination for self-achievement. With a diverse, challenging and progressive workout — each carefully customized session is designed to encourage the unity of mind, body and soul for a "complete body" experience. Teddy is more than just a trainer, he's a healer of souls. His reputation as a trainer is unsurpassed as he remains at the top of his field in its most competitive market — Los Angeles.

Teddy is a graduate of the University of North Carolina, Greensboro. He is a trained professional dancer and performer. He is featured regularly in a variety of fitness magazines and has been quoted in Allure, Cosmopolitan, In Style, Self and US Weekly to name a few. Connect with Teddy at TeddyBass.com.

Amika Ryan is a trainer, writer, rancher and mother. She has earned her MBA from Les Roches in Switzerland and her Certified Strength and Conditioning Specialist (CSCS®) credential. She specializes in physical rehabilitation, using a cooperative stretch therapy method, as a DCT™ Practitioner.

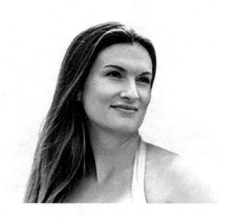

Amika lives in Montana with her daughter, Madison, and her dogs, Redmond and Coco. She enjoys shepherding her flock of Icelandic Sheep, and loves coming up with new ways to use their pelts, fleece and milk to make creative home and beauty products. Visit her at CopiaCove.com.

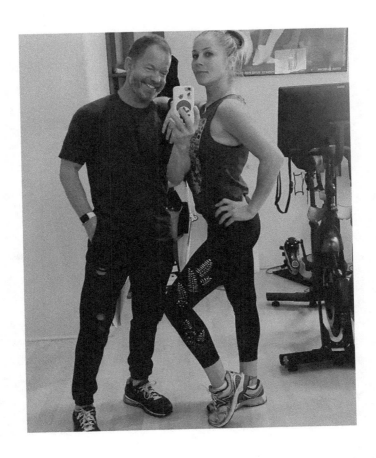

"Over 20 years ago I came to teddy after having a lot of personal issues that the effects had changed my body drastically. Teddy taught me that it was so much more than exercise. That holding on to emotional baggage had an even bigger effect on our health and fitness. This lesson he taught me has always stayed with me. He trains not only your body, but your mind and spirit as well. I Am so grateful to have him in my life. And so proud of his journey that has brought him to this book!! Bravo my sweet friend!"

- Christina Applegate, Award-winning Actress

— 1 —
BODY

"The body is your temple.
Keep it pure and clean for the soul to reside in."
— B.K.S. Iyengar

"The body is a sacred garment."
— Martha Graham

NUTRITION

Eat with One Thing on Your Mind

Eat Real Breakfast

Make the Fresh Choice

Snack Healthy or Not At All

K.I.S.S. with Simple Swaps

Drink Up

Do Caffeine Right

Catch Some Rays

Take a Multivitamin

Regularly Release (Your Bowels)

Eat with One Thing on Your Mind

What is your relationship with food? Have you eaten an entire pint of ice cream or bag of chips without realizing it? Do you eat in the car or while you check your phone? Do you eat when you are not physically hungry? We consume 30 percent more when we are distracted while eating, and not focused on eating while we are eating. That's a lot of unneeded and under appreciated calories.

Emotional and unconscious eating contributes to the obesity rate in our country and has fueled the popularity of fast food chains and unhealthy packaged, processed foods. Food should be used for your body to obtain energy and vital nutrients, and should be eaten consciously. The first step to changing unhealthy habits is to bring your awareness to them. Be more aware of how you are eating. Eating should be pleasurable and mindful at the same time, and immediate gratification needs to be taken out of the equation.

It's difficult, I get it! Personally, I have a single-parent, multi-tasking, ultra-social, operating system. I am always reminding myself to breathe and express gratitude in stillness before I eat.

Food journaling is a great tool that will bring your awareness to how you were feeling, or what you were doing, while you were eating. It is time to free yourself from the emotional hold that food has on you. And remember, inevitably, you are what you eat!

Take Action: Eat your meals mindfully. Take five deep breaths before this meal. Chew each bite 20 times. Eat until you are 80 percent full. And do nothing else but eat - no TV, no phone, no distractions. Remember, it takes twenty minutes for the brain to signal you are full. Slow down! Start by doing this with one meal per day, and work your way up to all meals.

<u>AFFIRMOTION</u>

Today, I choose to be present while eating, bringing my awareness to each meal. I make conscious choices for foods that support my efforts to be fit and healthy, moment-to-moment.

Eat Real Breakfast

You may not always feel like having breakfast, but, in my opinion, it is the most important meal of the day. Think of eating breakfast like you are fueling a machine as it begins its daily tasks. You cannot drive your car anywhere on "E", or without being fully charged. Eat what makes you feel good and fuels your engine, so that you can function at your highest potential. Start your day by setting the bar high for your nutritional uptake and reinforcing mindful eating habits.

Coffee and a pastry for breakfast will set you up for a blood sugar crash after the initial caffeine and sugar high. If you must have coffee in the morning, include some healthy fat while you are having the coffee, not after, to create lasting energy and feelings of satisfaction and well-being. Try whole nuts and seeds or their butters: almond butter or tahini are good choices.

It is always the best option (and I repeat, the best option) to sit down and eat whole foods for breakfast. Excellent breakfast foods to incorporate into your meal that pack a healthy-fat punch are avocados, olives, coconut, eggs, and wild salmon. Aim for 30 grams of protein, too, for optimal muscle synthesis. Great protein-rich foods are eggs, beans, greek yogurt, nuts and nut butters.

Breakfast smoothies are a great go-to on busy mornings when you may not have time to make a wholesome breakfast and sit down to eat. You can change it up with different berries, butters, or milks. Just make sure you are adding a quality protein powder. You get bonus points for adding a green powder or handful of leafy greens, which have valuable fiber, vitamins and minerals. Try adding a pinch of cinnamon to your breakfast to balance your blood sugar.

Take Action: Allow five more minutes for your morning routine and devote those minutes to breakfast. Spend five more minutes with your breakfast, either by making it, enjoying it, or sitting down to eat it. You might need to set your alarm clock five minutes earlier so that you have this extra time!

AFFIRMOTION

I choose to fuel this vessel of mine with nutrient-dense foods so that my mind and body get a great start each morning. I'm propelled into my day with clarity, vitality, and vigor!

Make the Fresh Choice

Keep your food choices fresh and organic. Shop the outside perimeter of your local market where you will find the fresh produce, dairy and meats. Buying fresh and organic can be more expensive, but it is higher quality food and more nutritious.

Common sense leads us to believe that anything with the word "fresh" in it must be better for us than anything packaged. This is true for the most part, but have you ever wondered why? Fresh to me means that the food is living and will naturally go bad, leaving out the chemical preservatives, and the nutritional value is considerably higher than packaged foods. Eating more fresh fruits and vegetables not only improves your health and moods, but your overall well-being as well.

Shop the outside aisles of your grocery store more often, even if it is a bit cooler around the outside. This helps burn more calories anyway because your body has to expend energy to keep you warm, so don't be shy. Avoid most of the center and frozen food aisles, and you will save yourself the chemicals found in many canned, processed and frozen foods. Try to incorporate these fresh and raw foods into every meal.

Certain types of organic produce can reduce the amount of toxins you consume on a daily basis by as much as 80 percent, according to the Environmental Working Group. This ultimately reduces your risk of cancer and other diseases. That sounds pretty important.

Take Action: Need some ideas on how to incorporate more fresh foods into your meals? Add a handful of greens to your eggs or smoothie in the morning or try some berries with a handful of raw nuts for a healthy snack. Keep it organic!

AFFIRMOTION

I take the time to shop for fresh produce and prepare healthy and nutritious meals for myself and my family. I allow the food I eat to fuel my creative desire to live this life to my fullest potential.

Snack Healthy or Not At All

When you think snacks, do you think donuts, candy bars, cookies, or potato chips? If so, your snack food cabinet probably needs a healthy upgrade. Choosing great tasting snacks that are fast, easy, and better for you is a win-win-win. They will help stabilize your blood sugar throughout the day, which translates to better moods, more energy, and stabilized weight. Here are some better snack options for you to swap:

- Elevate your apple with a tablespoon of almond butter.
- Ditch the cocoa chocolate bar for raw chocolate with 70-80% cacao.
- Avoid the pastry and grab some dried fruit with a handful of nuts, instead.
- Dance away from the party mix and grab some sprouted hummus with gluten free pretzels.
- Shy away from big-brand jerkies and go for low-sodium, all-natural, and gluten-free beef, turkey, or salmon jerky.
- Skip the potato chips and head for the bean chips with salsa.

In addition, when you think about snacks, make sure you think fresh, alive/raw, and green. Think, a wide variety of fruits and vegetables. Processed and preserved foods in bags, bottles, boxes, or cans have no place in a healthy diet.

Take Action: Today, have two healthy snacks. Eat one snack between breakfast and lunch, and the second snack between lunch and dinner. Notice any changes in your energy level or mood.

AFFIRMOTION

I easily find myself preparing healthy snacks that provide me with energy, empower me, and contribute to my longevity. I am productive, energized, and at my peak throughout the day.

K.I.S.S. with Simple Swaps

Keep it Simple, Swaps (KISS)! Simple swaps can really help ease you into a healthier lifestyle, rather than trying to quit your unhealthy habits cold-turkey. Try some of these simple switch-a-roos to boost your health IQ:

- Drink smoothies instead of soda.
- Swap artificial sweeteners for stevia, agave, xylitol, or honey.
- Swap out your sweet treat for organic dark chocolate or cacao.
- Focus on what you want instead of what you do not want.
- Walk or bike instead of drive.
- Swap out refined grains (white flour) for whole grains.
- Eat fresh seasonal foods instead of preserved and processed foods.

You can do this!

Take Action: Make a two-column list with headings "unhealthy" and "healthy". Write down all of the unhealthy items or habits you would like to change on the left side. Next to each "unhealthy" item, write down your "healthy" swap-out item on the right side. Start implementing these healthy swaps at a pace that is comfortable for you.

<u>AFFIRMOTION</u>

I easily find myself selecting healthier and more satisfying foods that fully nourish my body, support my mind, and sustain my energy level throughout the day.

Drink Up

Water is your body's principal chemical component, making up about 75 percent of it. Every system in your body depends on water. Water flushes toxins out of vital organs, carries nutrients to your cells and provides a moist environment for ear, nose, and throat tissues.

Lack of water can lead to dehydration, a condition that occurs when you don't have enough water in your body to carry out normal functions. Even mild dehydration can drain your energy and make you tired. Living in Los Angeles, where it can get very hot and dry, I am always toting around my water container!

Not all water is created equal. Make sure you are hydrating with quality water that is purified, mineralized, and alkaline. Follow these guidelines for optimal hydration:

- Drink at least one liter of water for every 50 pounds of body weight.
- Purify your water. Purifying water takes out impurities, but also essential minerals.
- Add back the minerals using trace mineral drops so that water can be delivered back into your body's cells.
- Increase the alkalinity of your water by adding a slice of lemon. Alkaline water is great because it keeps your body pH balanced.
- Coconut water will rehydrate you by replacing your body's needed fluids and electrolytes.
- Limit carbonated water, as it thins the lining of the gut.
- Drink water out of a non-leaching plastic, metal, or glass container.

Take Action: Go to your local health food store and pick up a bottle of Trace Mineral Drops to add to your water. You can also have your tap water analyzed for purity. If you're not sure your water is a safe and great candidate for hydration, invest in a good water filter.

<u>AFFIRMOTION</u>

I choose to drink water optimized for my best health and which promotes my best self. My body receives the balance of minerals it needs to be hydrated throughout the day.

Do Caffeine Right

Is caffeine your friend or enemy? No doubt, caffeine can give you energy and help you focus, but there are drawbacks to habitual use. The temporary fix provides instant energy, but also creates a stress-hormone response. Ultimately, this drains you, and prolonged caffeine abuse can set you up for adrenal problems in the future.

Caffeine can affect your mental health as well, by contributing to anxiety. For me, caffeine consumption jacks me up so much that I become hyperactive, want to run a marathon, resulting in me being much less productive. Caffeine also weakens your immune system by leaching vitamins and minerals, and it is dehydrating.

If you must have coffee, I recommend just having a cup in the morning. By no means should you be caffeinating after 12pm, as this can cause sleep disturbances. That being said, if you are going to drink coffee, make sure you are not using a plastic cup and that your coffee is organic. Add additional water to your coffee. Adequate water will reduce headaches, cravings and fatigue. You can also chew cardamom seeds to sweeten coffee breath, and help reduce the acidic effects of coffee on your stomach.

Take Action: Take an inventory of your caffeine intake. Caffeine doesn't just come from coffee. You can get it from energy drinks, teas, cocoa beans (chocolate), sodas, decaf coffee and some pain relievers (particularly for migraines). Where can you cut back? If you are habitually hooked on caffeine, maybe start cutting back by having just one cup of coffee a day.

<u>AFFIRMOTION</u>

I am full of energy and enthusiasm, naturally. I have an excess of stamina to make every day a great day.

Catch Some Rays

Vitamin D has been a hot topic for a while now because so many people are deficient. Vitamin D boosts bone health, helps fight against colds and elevates your mood. Deficiency is a leading cause of mild to moderate depression, and contributes to many other minor to serious health conditions.

You need at least 20 minutes of sunlight per day to get an optimal level of vitamin D. Doctors recommend a daily vitamin D supplement for most people. You may even need a prescription high-dose of vitamin D from your doctor to correct your levels if you are severely deficient. Sun makes for a healthier life, but make sure to use sunscreen, I recommend using a broad spectrum sunscreen with a SPF between 25 and 50, or cover up as needed to prevent damaging, and potentially cancer-causing, rays and burning.

Even people in sunny California, like myself, should be screened annually for vitamin D levels. You can check your vitamin D levels with a blood panel, or there are in-home test kits available. The normal range of vitamin D is 20 to 50 ng/mL, but an optimal functioning vitamin D level is over 60 ng/mL. Lower than 60ng/mL and you are at increased risk of depression, brain fog, skin problems, and other health problems.

These few minutes under the sun each day can literally change your life.

Take Action: Get outside (remember to bring cover-ups and sunscreen) and get more sun, or take a daily vitamin D supplement with a healthy meal or fish oil. Vitamin D is fat-soluble, and doing this will increase absorption.

AFFIRMOTION

I receive the benefits the universe provides for me from the sun and vitamin D. The benefits are here for me to accept and enjoy, and I do so gratefully.

Take a Multivitamin

It's good to cover all of your nutritional bases by taking a multivitamin, especially if you are not under the regular care of a nutritionist. First, have a blood panel performed by your healthcare professional to identify deficiencies. Keep in mind that normal levels are not the same as levels for optimal health.

Adding a multivitamin supplement is a no-brainer for most of us because it will cover all of your basic nutritional requirements. This is especially true if you are not confident that you are getting all the nutrients you need from eating a variety of fresh foods.

Consider supplementing with vitamin D as well, as it is the number one vitamin deficiency in the United States. Sublingual administration of Vitamin D is best for optimal absorption.

Rounding out the list of basic supplements to consider are fish oil for a healthy heart, probiotics for a healthy gut, and greens (containing spirulina, chlorella, and sea vegetables) for removing toxins.

Take Action: Upgrade your daily multivitamin to one that is a food-based, high-quality multivitamin. Ask your doctor or nutritionist for a recommendation. This might be the added boost you've been needing!

AFFIRMOTION

I make proactive health choices that are right for my body. I set myself up for optimal performance, and safeguard my future health.

Regularly Release (Your Bowels)

Your mind isn't the only part of your body that needs to release and let go in order for you to thrive. Your bowels do as well!

Your gut health and bowel movements are important because, when optimized, a healthy digestive system will help you live longer. It breaks down and delivers nutrients to your body and is also the most natural and healthy way to eliminate toxins from your body. There are many ways you can support your digestive system from the moment it goes in, to the point when it comes out.

Eating mindfully gives your digestive system a head start toward breaking down nutrients in your food. Remember, as I stated earlier, do not do anything else while you are eating (like watch TV, text or drive). Slow down, chew each bite of food thoroughly, breathe deeply, and notice how your food looks, tastes, smells, and feels.

As you get older, stomach acid declines, contributing to indigestion and other health problems. You need stomach acid to break down protein and destroy pathogens in your gut. Supplementing with betaine hydrochloride can support digestive function when taken with meals, by increasing stomach acid. You can take betaine HCL along with a digestive enzyme to help break down foods further and extract the maximum amount of nutrients.

To promote regular bowel movements, be sure that you are drinking sufficient water. Eat fibrous foods, such as whole grains, nuts, fresh fruits, vegetables and beans. Taking a multi-strain probiotic, or eating foods with natural probiotics in them such as live-cultured yogurt and fermented foods, like keifer, kombucha tea, miso, kimchi, and sauerkraut, will keep your gut in tip top shape. And you may wish to invest in a squatty-potty, which puts you in a better anatomical position to produce effortless number twos.

Take Action: Evaluate your digestive health. Are you having less than one bowel movement per day? Do you strain to produce a bowel movement? Do you have gas or bloating? Do you have bad breath? Do you have trouble losing weight? If you answered yes to any of these questions, try some of the tips above to improve your digestive health. After all, you don't want to be needlessly hanging onto anything that could weigh you down!

AFFIRMOTION

I easily allow movement to happen in all areas of my life. My body operates at a high level of efficiency and grace, digesting and releasing effortlessly.

HEALTHCARE

Ensure You're Insured

Your Hearty Heart

Take Care of Those Tootsies

Brush Floss Smile

Wash Your Hands

Ensure You're Insured

Until recently, over 40 million people in the United States did not have healthcare because they either could not afford it, or just did not think they needed it. Since the Affordable Healthcare Act, many more Americans are able to obtain coverage for medical expenses.

Make sure you have healthcare coverage that is appropriate for your needs. Personally, having the security of medical coverage for me and my family, far outweighs the monthly payments that I make for that coverage. I'm certainly not counting on having a sudden medical emergency, but I am prepared in case anything does happen.

Take Action: Evaluate your current health insurance with a professional. Be sure you have coverage that works best for you financially, and that you are covered now for possible situations in the future.

<u>AFFIRMOTION</u>

I am informed and involved in maintaining my best option in healthcare coverage for myself and my family. I make wise decisions concerning my health, wealth, and well being.

Your Hearty Heart

Your diet and lifestyle directly affect blood quality, the health of the blood vessels, and your heart. According to the Centers for Disease Control and Prevention (CDC), heart disease remains the leading cause of death in the United States. This statistic alone should open your eyes to the importance of heart health. You are at risk of atherosclerosis (plaque build-up in blood vessels) if you have a family history of heart disease, smoke, are sedentary, obese, have high blood pressure, diabetic, and/or chronically stressed. Heart disease is preventable in most cases, and is largely affected by your daily lifestyle choices and diet.

To keep your heart beating strong:

- Exercise at least 30 minutes every day with the goal of elevating your heart rate.

- Reduce inflammation by avoiding gluten, dairy, sugar, and alcohol in your diet and avoid any other environmental or food allergens as these cause inflammation too.

- Get more antioxidants into your diet from berries, beets, red bell pepper, brussels sprouts and kale. Support your body's fat metabolism by getting more coconut oil, radish, green onion, and leeks in your diet.

- Manage your stress with yoga, meditation, or breathing exercises.

- Absolutely no smoking.

You can also supplement your diet with vitamin B-12 and fish oil to support a healthy cardiovascular system. Insufficient B-12 levels can lead to a higher risk of heart disease. Vitamin B-12 is particularly difficult to absorb as you age, so go for the sublingual supplement for best results. The omega-3s in fish oil thin the blood, and are needed for maintaining blood pressure and regulating cholesterol. A fish oil supplement is recommended if you are not eating wild, fatty fish three times a week.

Take Action: What habits can you change to give your heart some extra love? Choose one right now and commit to doing that one thing - quit smoking, go for a 30 minute walk every morning, take up an active stress-relieving activity, or kick all alcohol and sugar to the curb! If not now, when? You are your own best advocate for your vitality.

<u>AFFIRMOTION</u>

I make daily choices to keep myself moving, grooving, giving, and laughing. I consider all aspects of my life when supporting my heart to beat strong and be vibrant.

Take Care of Those Tootsies

You will travel more than 75,000 miles on your feet by age 50! And I bet that I, have done more miles than that already!

Your feet are the foundation upon which your body is built, and moves you through life. Unhealthy feet can throw your entire body out of balance, which is a recipe for chronic pain.

Make sure your feet have good circulation. Tight shoes, high heels, cold temperatures, and standing for long periods of time can reduce blood circulation to your feet. Make sure your shoes fit correctly and that you are moving around often. If you sit at a desk all day, take your shoes off and use a golf ball to gently massage your feet.

Take Action: Consider going to a pedorathist or podiatrist, both foot experts, to determine if you need orthotics. Even if you have perfectly healthy feet, the periodic use of orthotics can be extremely beneficial. For example, if you carry heavy weight like a backpack for an extended period of time, or stand for long periods of time at your job, you may benefit from orthotics.

AFFIRMOTION

I have healthy and beautiful feet. I am grateful that they carry me steadily through all of my adventures in this life.

Brush Floss Smile

Remember the last conversation you had with someone where you could not wait for it to be over because of either your, or their, bad breath? There are few things worse than talking with someone that has halitosis! It is important to practice good oral hygiene, because the health of your mouth reflects the health of your entire body and leaves a good impression.

Having your teeth cleaned regularly and brushing and flossing after meals have been proven to reduce cavities, thereby reducing dental healthcare costs for fillings, the possibility of needing false teeth, root canals, and bridges as you age -- all of which are undesirably expensive and painful. Having a healthy mouth will also boost your self-confidence. You'll smile more, and we all know that smiling and laughter are great for your health.

Take Action: Call your dentist and make an appointment if you have not had your teeth cleaned within the last six months.

AFFIRMOTION

Good oral hygiene is a priority in my life. I honor myself by flossing and brushing thoroughly at least twice daily.

Wash Your Hands

"Cleanliness is next to godliness" is what I grew up hearing. All day long we are putting our hands on surfaces that contain bacteria and viruses -- surfaces like escalators, counters, tables, chairs, toilets, doors, gym equipment, and toys. You expose your body to these germs by putting your hands in your mouth, or by touching your eyes or nose.

Removing germs through washing your hands frequently during the day helps prevent diarrhea and respiratory infections, and may even help prevent skin and eye infections. This is doubly important in my household, where it seems that my son brings home twice as many germs as any other kid!

I hope you know how to properly wash your hands by now, but here is a reminder:

- Wet your hands with clean, running water (warm or cold), turn off the tap, and apply soap.
- Lather your hands and be sure to get the backs of your hands, between your fingers, and under your nails.
- Scrub your hands for at least 20 seconds.
- Rinse your hands well under running water.
- Dry your hands completely using a clean towel, or completely air-dry them.
- Use the towel to turn off the tap.

Wash your hands frequently. It is recommended that you and your family wash your hands before and after preparing food, before eating food, before and after being around someone who may be sick, after using the bathroom, changing diapers, blowing your nose, sneezing, coughing, touching garbage, and after handling pets or pet food.

I am not a huge fan of using the antibacterial hand gels. They can be harmful if swallowed, burn your eyes, and have been proven to contribute to antibiotic resistance. Instead, I recommend using an all-natural hand sanitizer. You will avoid the parabens, triclosan, and chemicals found in the gels. Keep it in your car or purse, and use as needed.

Take Action: Make your own all-natural hand sanitizer. Mix two parts 100 percent aloe vera, two parts witch hazel (without alcohol), one part apple cider vinegar, and several drops of an antibacterial essential oil, like lavender or clove, in a small spray bottle. Shake before each use.

AFFIRMOTION

I show myself great respect through excellent hygiene habits, and these habits benefit my overall well being.

EXERCISE

Move It and Gain It

Go Outside

Be Flexible to Explore

Workout Smarter, Not Harder

Exercise for Life

The Core Component of Fitness

Move It and Gain It

One of my favorite sayings that I've created over my years as a trainer is, "Move it and lose it!" In this case, it is more appropriately stated, "Move it and gain it!" - muscle and strength, that is. Physical exercise and nutrition are the key components to maintaining and gaining strength.

Movement is crucial to your strength, good health and well-being. No one is asking you to train like an Olympic athlete, but regular exercise is a must. You need a minimum of 30 minutes of a combination of aerobic and resistance exercises three days a week to combat muscle loss as you get older.

Make sure you have an adequate intake of protein of 100 grams per day. Protein deficiency can cause decreased muscle mass, fatigue and mental fog. Choose foods that are rich in high-quality protein, such as fish, eggs, dairy, poultry, and lamb. Nuts, seeds, and beans contain protein as well -- just keep in mind that these are not as concentrated as animal sources of protein.

Take Action: Working out should be fun, so move your body in ways you enjoy. If yoga is not for you, then don't force it. Find an activity that you enjoy: dance, swim, play tennis or golf (sitting doesn't count)! This will make exercising seem less like work and more like fun.

<u>AFFIRMOTION</u>

I easily find myself doing thirty minutes of cardiovascular or strength building exercise each day, enhancing my physical and mental well-being. I am committed to living a long, prosperous, and healthy life.

Go Outside

John Muir said, "Everybody needs beauty as well as bread, places to play in and pray in, where nature may heal and give strength to body and soul alike." Spend time outside in fresh air. Appreciate nature. Choose to walk outside, walk your dog, or play with your kids outside. Being in nature brings to each of us the gift of appreciation.

Doing activities outdoors not only helps burn calories, but changes your environment and keeps you motivated. This new scene will give you a new perspective. Get outside and get moving!

Take Action: While outside, keep a lookout for tools you can use for added fitness challenges. A bench, for example, can be used for squats, dips, or even as a step-up. Use a line on the ground as a marker for side-to-side hops. Or use the mailbox at the end of the street as your goal for distance.

AFFIRMOTION

I easily accept the bounty of love, light, and energy that nature has to give me. I let it flow through my entire being as I actively participate in my life.

Be Flexible to Explore

Flexibility is perhaps the most overlooked aspect of a well-balanced fitness program. As a refresher, key components of any physical fitness program includes strength training, cardiovascular exercise, core strength, balance, and flexibility. Maintaining flexibility becomes increasingly more difficult as you age. You may find stretching less enjoyable, and not do it as much as it becomes more challenging, thus contributing to even more lack of flexibility.

It doesn't matter if you can't even remember the last time you stretched. All the more reason to start right now! Be consistent, and you'll soon see improvements in your range of motion and feel the benefits of a reduction in your stress level. This should keep you motivated to keep going.

There are many ways to stretch. If you are not finding yoga enjoyable anymore, try a stretching or martial arts class. Martial arts are also great for improving your balance, which helps prevent accidents, such as falls. Any new activity that includes stretching before or after, would do the trick as well. There are also some different stretch philosophies that you can explore, like fascial stretching and foam rolling.

The goal is to at least maintain a functional range of motion, and balance, in order to safely perform your normal activities.

Take Action: Explore a new way to stretch. Schedule yourself in a class this week that is either all about stretching, or incorporates several minutes of stretching into the program.

<u>AFFIRMOTION</u>

I easily incorporate more breathing, flexibility, and stretching into my day. I embrace calm and relaxation everywhere at anytime.

Workout Smarter, Not Harder

Tune in and pay attention to your body, how it feels, and what it is telling you. Make sure you take time to rest before you are exhausted. Pushing past our comfortable tired limit not only can lead to burn-out and physical injuries, but can also stress you hormonally, leading to sleep disorders, weight gain, inability to lose weight, and digestive issues.

When it comes to working out, drop the "no pain no gain" way of thinking. You may have been told or heard somewhere that if you are not in pain then you are not working hard enough. This is the very reason why 65 percent of people who start working out stop before they have reached the six-month milestone. It's better to exercise smarter, not harder.

My rule of thumb is, start easy at a pace that feels good for you, where you can remain consistent. Then, gradually begin to increase the intensity and duration of your workouts. You will see a difference within weeks. Your body will start to desire the endorphins and natural energy that are produced from your sustainable efforts. You will look forward to your exercise and avoid any of the negative effects of over-stressing your system.

Everybody is different when it comes to his or her comfortable stress limit. Make sure you are on a sustainable workout schedule that energizes you, and that you look forward to doing.

Take Action: On days or weeks that you are particularly stressed from work or whatever else is going on in your life, decrease the intensity of your exercise session. This gives your body a better a chance of recovering from the hormonal stresses you are experiencing, without the added stress of a taxing workout.

<u>AFFIRMOTION</u>

I am in tune with my body. I make choices that support my physical and emotional well-being. I create harmony and vigor.

Exercise for Life

It is a good idea for everyone to learn how to move in the way that the human body is designed to move. We all used to have the perfect squat form. Just look at any toddler pick something up off the ground. As adults, most of us have forgotten how our bodies are designed to hinge and angle to move.

Stationary movements on an exercise machine, or even with dumbbells, limit your range of motion and inhibit the use of multiple joints. These do not resemble many functional daily movements, and have little additional benefits other than building isolated muscle mass. There is a more beneficial and efficient way to move called functional exercise.

Functional exercises have many benefits, such as burning more calories and keeping your heart rate up. These types of exercises can even spare you from possible injury during everyday tasks.

Think of functional exercise as movements that mimic everyday motions that you regularly perform. For example, the squat is probably the most common movement that humans use (or should use, anyway). Have you heard people say, "Lift with your legs, not your back?" They are telling you to "squat." The squat uses your hips and legs - the largest and most powerful muscle groups - to do the heavy lifting, while your back remains in a safe and stable position with an engaged core.

Stop sitting and start moving!

Take Action: Use more multi-joint movements in your workouts. Try adding functional movements like the squat-to-press, lunge-and-twist, and even burpees. You can also upgrade movements that you may already be doing. For example, if you are doing a standing biceps curl, upgrade to an underhand pull-up, and then move yourself right down into a push up.

AFFIRMOTION

I incorporate multi-joint exercises into my routine that allow my body to stay strong. I perform everyday, functional motions with awareness, comfort, and ease.

The Core Component of Fitness

Core strength is one of the most overused terms in the fitness industry today. It is also one of the most important factors in a balanced, healthy body. This core component of fitness is important because your deep abdominal and back muscles work together to stabilize your spine, keeping your back injury and pain free, improving your balance, and making every whole-body movement you perform more effective.

Choose to incorporate exercises in each workout to specifically strengthen your core muscles. Planks are great for strengthening your transverse abdominals and lower back extensors. Perform the side plank exercise to target your obliques. And the hip bridge is a great exercise for your glutes and increases functional integration, the "working together", of your posterior chain (back, glutes, and hamstrings). You are also activating your core muscles while doing whole body movements, like the squat, lunge, and deadlift.

Remember to start out easy and work your way up in time or repetitions as your body adapts to these exercises.

Take Action: Do a core strengthening series each day this week consisting of 30 second holds of six hip bridges, three side planks (each side), and four planks. Adjust your numbers of repetitions or time in the hold as needed.

<u>AFFIRMOTION</u>

My core is strong and resilient. I am conscious of these muscles and their unwavering support, and continue to incorporate core strengthening exercises into my health routine.

SELF CARE

You Need to be Kneaded

Press Pause

Make Time for Intimacy

Toxin-Free Please

Give Yourself a Reward: Vacation

Sleep Baby Sleep

You Need to be Kneaded

Self-care and touch are important parts of being in tune with your body. When you are aware of the physical signals your body is sending you, then you can be prepared to fight off possible sickness, injuries, discomfort, and mood swings. Give yourself permission to slow down, and take some time for your body to recover. It is amazing what a little quiet time can do for your mind, body, and soul.

There are many ways to release your body tension and promote healing through bodywork. For example, there is nothing better than a spa day to help you relax and pamper yourself. Use the hot tub, sauna, and shower to loosen tense muscles. Getting a massage is great for working out the kinks in your muscles (and the best part is that someone else is doing all the work). If a regular massage is not in your budget and money is an issue, stretch your body out on a foam roller, or even watch a YouTube video and do some stretches at home. Take a hot bath in epsom salt, sea salt, and baking soda, or a long, hot shower!

Whether you are a do-it-yourselfer or employing a professional, remember to take deep breaths to get maximum benefits. Unplug regularly from the world at large. And yes, that means shutting off your phone, computer and television, too!

Take Action: Block out an hour once a week for bodywork that focuses on releasing your tension area(s) and stretching tight muscles. Or, take an hour daily to quiet your phone and computer and take a break from the bombardment of social media, texts, calls and emails. You deserve it, and your body will feel a whole lot better.

AFFIRMOTION

I allow myself time to rest, relax, and connect with my body. I am more productive in my daily activities, and embrace a more relaxed and peaceful self.

Press Pause

It is important for you to take a few moments each day to press pause, slow down, and let everything sink in. Notice the sounds and smells around you. Feel your heart beat, and notice your breath. It may be hard for you at first, but practice, practice, practice, and you'll soon realize amazing benefits from being more mindful.

You may need to set a reminder on your phone, or you can start as simply as taking five breaths every time you start your car. Adding this to your daily awareness practice will give you a more positive outlook on life, lower your blood pressure, and help you be more clear-headed and more appreciative. Here are some other ideas to promote your mindfulness:

- Wake up slow and remember your dreams.
- Give thanks before you eat a meal.
- Take the long way to your car in the parking lot and enjoy being outside.
- Light candles before you start to cook dinner.

Many of us are always on the go, with the goal of being more productive and keeping busy. The truth is, you will probably get more done and be more efficient and clear-headed if you take the time to slow down. Studies have shown that practicing being mindful will allow you to be more focused.

Take Action: Take ten minutes each day, starting now, to breathe and be still (or meditate). This is your sacred time to be quiet and let the mind slow down. Let all your thoughts drift away like bubbles floating on a breeze. You can work your way up to 30 minutes, as you get accustomed to the practice. After, your mind will be clearer and this is a great time to recognize your healthy desires and set intentions for your life goals.

AFFIRMOTION

I am a person who easily presses pause to center my mind, allowing myself to be more present and responsive in my daily life.

Make Time for Intimacy

Does your sex-life need a jump-start? If yes, I have great news for you. Improving your health is a great reason to have more sex. It has been proven to increase good feelings, decrease bad feelings, and even prevent cancer.

The release of oxytocin during and after sex leads to better and longer sleep, increased marital satisfaction, and greater feelings of overall happiness. Sex also relieves stress by decreasing the stress hormone cortisol. It has also been proven that men who have more sex have less chance of getting prostate cancer.

Sex also brings you intimacy and connection, which always feels good. Ensure you have a healthy sex-life by keeping the lines of communication open with your partner. Or, if you do not have a partner at this time, keep your self-connection alive!

Partnerships and marriages go through patches where lack of sex may be part of the problem. Be willing to communicate with your partner about what is working for you sexually, and ask often about their needs, too. Trust, communication, and respect set the foundation for healthy, connected relationships, as well as your sex relationship with your partner.

Remember, you can still cash in on many of the benefits sex has to offer even if you are only having sex with yourself.

Take Action: Sometimes it's hard to find time for sex, but individuals and couples who schedule time for sex have more sex than people who do not. Get with your partner (or yourself) and pencil (read: permanent marker) some lovemaking into the calendar.

AFFIRMOTION

I am a desirable being. I choose and desire healthy and positive connections.

Toxin-Free Please

Make label-reading part of your regular reading list. From shampoo to lotion, and from deodorant to makeup, you need to be educated about what you put on your body. What is best for you is not always what is being sold to you, contrary to the fancy packaging and advertisements. This is important because what you put on your body affects your health -- just as much as what you eat.

Your body consumes or absorbs everything it touches through the skin, eyes, nose, and mouth. It only takes 26 seconds for these products to enter your bloodstream. What does your body come into contact with on a daily basis? Lotions, hair care products, household cleaners, detergents, fragrances, makeup? These products can contain toxic chemicals that may make you sick. These chemicals have been linked to cancer, skin problems, headaches, inflammation, reproductive problems, eye damage, and chronic fatigue, in addition to other health problems. Products are not regulated by, or forced to comply with, many safety standards.

Although there are potentially several different toxins in any one home or beauty product, these are the top four to definitely avoid:

- DEA (diethanolamine), a wetting and foaming agent found in shampoos, soaps, and detergent, is linked to cancer.

- Sodium laurel/lareth sulfate is a skin irritant with corrosive properties that was originally designed as a pesticide with corrosive properties.

- Propylene glycol, also found in and latex paint and anti-freeze, decreases fertility.

- Paraben (petroleum byproduct) causes early puberty because it mimics estrogen, and also contributes to breast cancer.

Educate yourself on the dangers that may be hiding in your beauty and cleaning products, and take responsibility for your health. Environmental Working Group is a great resource that rates the safety of products. You can check it out online at ewg.org.

Take Action: Take the most common product you put on your skin, and read the ingredients on the label. Does it contain anything you would not eat, or cannot explain or pronounce? It might be time to think about a new favorite. Give yourself permission to transition slowly, as this can be an expensive replacement process. Pick one or two products a week, and repeat.

AFFIRMOTION

I easily take a few moments to remove products that no longer serve me, and select those that are safest and healthiest for myself, my family, and my environment.

Give Yourself a Reward: Vacation

We all have stress in our lives. You may face the burden of meeting tight deadlines, making crucial decisions, or managing the complexities of household demands. It is easy to get caught up in these tasks and forget what a great job you are doing. Self-recognition, appreciation, and praise are key behaviors that help us to achieve continued success. Make it a priority to reward yourself for making progress toward your goals, no matter how small.

A vacation is arguably the ultimate reward. Planning a vacation will give you a deadline, and motivate you to get your work done so that you can sit back and relax. Shared family time, isolated from everyday activities, helps to promote positive relationships and lasting memories, as well as letting you decompress. You'll feel reenergized in no time.

Taking a vacation doesn't have to be expensive or time consuming. If you can't afford to get away because you have a tight budget or schedule, try doing a "stay-cation." Visit a local tourist attraction and bring a picnic. Turn off the electronics, do an at-home spa treatment, and light some candles. Pamper yourself. You deserve it. Taking care of yourself now makes you better able to handle stressful situations in the future.

Even if you have not met a particular goal, spend some time being grateful and honoring the progress toward that goal. That is a reward in itself because from this acceptance you will change and grow.

Take Action: Plan your next vacation or stay-cation. Mark a date on your calendar right now! Then, write about what you want to do, how you would like to feel, and what goals you want to accomplish before this date. Pick a destination or activity that will help you achieve your vision.

<u>AFFIRMOTION</u>

*As an active participant in my life,
I create time for relaxation and
rejuvenation. I am refreshed and present
in my own life.*

Sleep Baby Sleep

Have you ever suffered from insomnia or other sort of sleep disturbance? Over one-third of all people will be affected by insomnia at some point in their lives, according to the Mayo Clinic. Additionally, the National Sleep Foundation revealed studies stating that at least 40 million Americans suffer from over 70 different sleep disorders. These numbers are probably much higher since these statistics do not account for those not reported or diagnosed. I'm sure you can agree that sleep is essential for your health and well-being, and it seems that too many people are not getting enough quality sleep.

The amount of sleep needed per night varies from person to person. Some people can function perfectly on six, and others need as much as ten hours of sleep per night. It is important to get your magic number of hours per night, because you are missing out on physical and emotional healing if you do not. The first four hours of sleep contribute to your body's physical repair, and the remaining hours repair your brain and help you process emotions.

There are many reasons people cannot sleep, including those that are hormonal, diet, or lifestyle related. Solutions to your own sleep disturbances depend upon the cause. Here are my top six tips to help you get a better night's sleep. One, or a combination of them, will hopefully work for you.

- Stop Stimulants: No caffeine after 12pm. Skip the afternoon coffee, and go for a healthy snack instead.
- Stabilize Blood Sugar: Nuts before bed will help your blood sugar stay stable throughout the night.
- Boost Melatonin: Take a supplement or drink tart cherry juice. Stimulating melatonin production will help you fall asleep.

- Slow Down: Allow some transition time before bed.
- Relax: Sesame oil on the feet, and lavender oil to inhale, are sure to relax you before bed.
- Write a List: Jot down five things today you feel that could have gone better, and five things that really went your way! Feel gratitude for all ten things.

Take Action: Make room for quiet time 30 minutes before bed with no technology (TV, phone, tablet). Instead, spend that time stretching, reading for pleasure, just breathing, or jotting down a few things that worked, or didn't work, for you during the day.

If you are hooked on using your phone, switch the *night shift* setting to *on* to reduce the amount of blue light you are exposed to before bed. Blue light reduces melatonin production in your body, which is needed for sleep.

AFFIRMOTION

I accept the importance of sleep in my life. Its natural benefits restore my body and renew my mind. I fall asleep with ease.

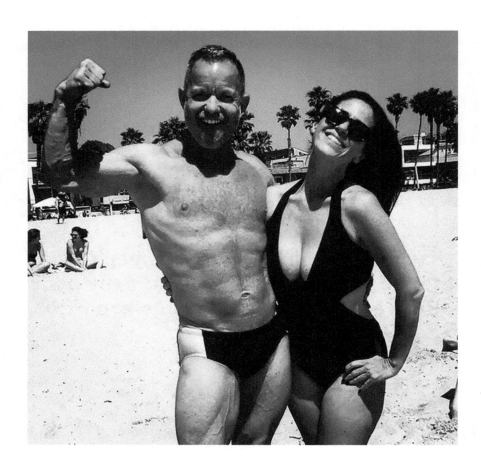

"I am so grateful to have Teddy in my life. I have worked out with him throughout the years. His dedication and inspiration have brought so much to my life. He is more than an incredible trainer. He is a teacher and a wonderful friend. He excepts me for me and I love him with all my heart. I can't wait to have this book with me as a constant reminder of him."

- Soleil Moon Frye, Actress, Director and Screenwriter

— 2 —
MIND

"My mission in life is not merely to survive, but to thrive; and to do so with some passion, some compassion, some humor, and some style."

— Maya Angelou

HEAD HEALTH

Don't Be List-less

Be A Goal Setter and Getter

Get Professional Help

Don't Be List-less

You are probably already familiar with the tool of making lists. They are a great way to keep your mind clutter-free and make sure you don't forget anything important. The most common excuse I hear from other parents or clients is, "Oh I forgot." Yes, I'm guilty as well, especially when my son asks me about something.

I give my son the excuse that I'm 42 years older than he is, and older people just forget more often than younger people. His suggestion? "Put it on your phone!" Without an ongoing list, as a single parent keeping up with his social and school schedule alone, I would go crazy. Organize yourself like I do by making a to-do list and revisit it daily. Have short and long-term tasks and chores that need to be completed, so the time sensitive things do not get lost in the shuffle.

Items can be something that you take care of right now, like "Make an appointment to see Dr. John," or months from now, like "Don't forget to pack your bathing suit." Essentially, anything that clears the clutter from your mind needs to go on a list. If you have something on your regular to-do list for more than a few weeks, it may need to go on a priority list.

List-keeping has helped me learn how to prioritize. It's handy to have it on my phone because I can access it wherever I am, changing things on the fly, and crossing things off as I do them. It is a great feeling of accomplishment to see the list get smaller and smaller. Revisit your lists often and prioritize.

Ask a friend for assistance in checking things off your list, if needed. The more the merrier!

Take Action: Make a fix-it list. Add all the things in your home or work space that need to be repaired, replaced, or finished; the things that nag at you, that need to get done but never seem to, that don't need to get done but drain your energy every time you see them. Write them down. Try to cross something off that list each day or each week. You'll feel lighter, more clear-headed, and energetic in no time.

AFFIRMOTION

This day I start with a breath. I meditate and allow the day to expand. I realize there is enough time and energy to do all the things that I have listed, with ease and grace.

Be A Goal Setter and Getter

We all need to have something to look forward to. What better way to keep ourselves accountable and to go after something that can change the course of our lives? Setting goals helps keep you focused and motivated. Having short-term, as well as long-term goals, is equally important to set for yourself because goals can help you prioritize your life and the things you want to accomplish.

You can think of short-term goals like having a bookmark. They will keep you focused and on track. Setting small, attainable goals is important for keeping your spirits up because you can celebrate often as you reach them. But don't be afraid to dream big, and to set huge goals, too.

Having long-term goals gives you a direction for your efforts that will pay off in the next five or ten years. They are like the North Star that guides your journey. Imagine the day when one of your big, long-term goals is finally achieved. There is nothing quite like it!

Take Action: Survey your current situation. Write down your short-term goals; a goal you will accomplish this week, this month and this year. Post this somewhere that you will see it every day. Be brave! You can even think long-term and add a 5 year goal.

AFFIRMOTION

My life is a constant upward spiral. I set goals that are attainable, realistic, tangible, timely, and rewarding to accomplish.

Get Professional Help

In my business, even with the professional certifications that I hold, I am not qualified to make diagnoses. So, I often refer to a professional who can help my client appropriately. You wouldn't go to a veterinarian to ask about a problem with your elbow. Don't procrastinate or self-diagnose -- get help from a professional. Professional health, life, or physical coaches can be great resources outside of your normal support circle.

It is important you find the right health professional with whom to work witt, that you trust, admire, and who inspires you. If you find someone that you are not 100 percent happy with, then find someone else. There are many different personalities, philosophies, and styles out there, and you are sure to have that important connection with someone. There is no need to limit yourself to somebody local. Video or audio conferences work just as well for many people as face-to-face meetings.

Some thoughts, experiences or dreams are best kept inside my professional network. From time to time, I need a little extra support in an area of my life, and can get it from my spiritual advisor. She is great when I need someone to listen to me and understand how I feel, without judgment. She is also able to notice, and point out patterns in my behavior that may be holding me back.

Take Action: Identify an area of your life that needs some extra TLC. Find a professional that will work one-on-one with you in this area. If money is an issue, talk with the professional about a plan that will work for both of you. The right person may be more flexible than you think. Also, there are many self-help books out there that you can read that may help you to take action in your life.

AFFIRMOTION

I am open to attract and receive professionals to help me in any area of my life that needs attention or support. Surrendering to assistance is empowering for me.

EMOTION

Let's Not Get Serious

Shake It Off

First, a Responder

Gratitude with Attitude

Laugh Out Loud, Often

Plant a Seed

Let's Not Get Serious

It seems like from an early age we are chomping at the bit to get older faster, by mastering and accomplishing more. Now that you have mastered and accomplished, back that pony up. Reverse the maturity-meter into something more blissfully innocent and childlike.

Having an optimistic, upbeat, and sometimes silly attitude leads to a happier life. You are never too old to be silly, start something new, or change your whole life. Life is too short to let your imagination be limited by the practicalities of being an adult. Foster your sense of humor, don't take things so seriously, and have more fun.

Take Action: Release the need to take yourself so seriously. Be silly and playful. Try singing your favorite song as if you were the original writer and performer, or whatever else that will allow you to feel light-hearted!

<u>AFFIRMOTION</u>

I integrate with my youthful spirit, celebrate my choice to live a light-hearted existence, and think positive thoughts often.

Shake It Off

Let it go and shake it off. Literally, don't let anything rain on your parade. It's okay to feel upset, angry, or frustrated because having and expressing emotions, good or bad, is normal and healthy. But be ready to let whatever it is go, once you have had time to process your emotions.

Firstly, make sure you are expressing your emotions rather than harboring emotions inside. Carrying around unexpressed emotions can be hazardous to your health. Sometimes you will need to scream, hit something, or cry. Make sure you are letting your emotions out in an appropriate setting (i.e. away from other people). Release them, and let go of the burden of carrying them around.

Remember, not everything is about you. We are meaning-making machines, but don't make something negative out of nothing at all. Be still, breathe, and stop concerning yourself with others and what they think about you. After all, people do not think about you as often as you think they do.

Lastly, forgive yourself. You are your own worst critic. Sometimes the voices in your head are more critical than anyone else around you. Recognize and start to quiet those voices. Make sure you are focusing instead on the unique gifts that you have, and do not be so hard on yourself.

Take Action: Is your internal negative self-talk getting you down? Quiet those voices, and extinguish their power by saying "I guess you could be right" and then ignoring them and moving on. Forgive yourself often - daily, hourly, and even every minute if needed. The only way to thrive is by removing the burdens, so let's get lifting.

AFFIRMOTION

Moment by moment, I am more aware of the thoughts that serve me and my highest good. I release all thoughts that limit me or keep me small.

First, A Responder

Are you reactive or responsive? We can all think of a situation where we spoke the first thing that popped into our head. Maybe you immediately regretted it, or maybe it was not a big deal. Either way, having the ability to respond to a situation rather than react without thought, can decrease your level of stress, make the best of a situation, and increase your quality of life.

Most of us think in terms of right or wrong, black and white, them and me, powerful or powerless. I am here to say that you have a choice about what you think. Become an observer of your own conversations and actions. The first step toward being able to appropriately respond is to notice when you are reacting.

Lao Tzu asked, "Do you have the patience to wait until your mud settles and the water is clear?" I think you do. Wait until your reaction has passed, and go from there. Everyone will benefit, especially you.

Allow your inner *responder* to show up in any conflict.

Take Action: Practice mindfulness to learn to respond. Notice when you react and take a moment, then let this moment pass. Think of what an appropriate response would be. Be kind to, and patient with yourself and others. Let go of shame, blame, and judgement.

AFFIRMOTION

With each breath, I easily connect to my inner calm and peaceful being, and respond in situations to everyone's highest good.

Gratitude with Attitude

Is your glass half-full or half-empty? Are you empathetic to others, or judgmental? Perspective is the one thing that is personal to each of us, but is also a choice. You can choose to be optimistic and understanding, instead of negative and critical.

Do not speak ill of another or judge. Simply take the high road, not to be superior, but to spread love and light to others. Try to empathize with others by seeing things from their point of view. You do not have to agree with them, but being able to appreciate where someone else is coming from will make for better social interactions.

It is all about perception. It helps to trust and know that you are going to be okay, no matter the outcome of a situation. That with which you are looking will determine what you see.

Take Action: Write a gratitude list. Include everything you are thankful for today, this week, this year -- whatever works best for you. Do this often to foster feelings of appreciation and happiness.

AFFIRMOTION

My attitude of gratitude opens doors for opportunities to flow into my life, and inspires me in all that I do.

Laugh Out Loud, Often

Don't take yourself too seriously. It adds to stress, tension, and judgment. A sure cure for the serious ones among us is laughter. Not only does laughter feel good while you are doing it, it's contagious, and has benefits that stretch beyond the moment.

Laughter boosts your immune system by activating t-cells, which helps fight off sickness. Other known benefits of laughing include decreasing stress hormones, releasing endorphins, and improving blood circulation and oxygen intake. In the end, you just feel awesome after a good hard laugh.

Take Action: Children are great generators of infectious laughter. If you don't have kids of your own, see if you can borrow a few from a friend. Take this opportunity to be silly, channel your inner child, and laugh a whole lot!

AFFIRMOTION

I easily allow my inner child to laugh out loud and feel the joy from within myself.

Plant A Seed

Did you know that having plants around you can improve your health and well being? Flowers, edible plants, and live decorative plants all provide great health benefits. Being around plants improves concentration, memory, and productivity, in addition to decreasing stress. Plants also purify the air around you.

Being around plants helps people concentrate better in the home and workplace. Having flowers around your home or office has been shown to greatly improve your mood and reduce the likelihood of stress-related depression. Flowers and ornamental plants increase levels of positive energy, to help you feel secure and relaxed. A recent University of Michigan study showed that the presence of plants can increase memory retention up to 20 percent. Nature in your home or workplace helps to stimulate your senses and your mind, which leads to improved mental cognition and performance. This research is also true for children. Being around plants helps kids concentrate and learn better, too.

Studies also show that people who spend time planting, growing, or caring for plants have less stress in their lives. Plants can provide a positive way for you to convert your stress into nurturing. Spending more time around plants will also make you more likely to try and help others, and often leading to more advanced social relationships.

Plants are also good for the air you breathe. Through photosynthesis, plants absorb carbon dioxide and release oxygen. More oxygen in your home means a better functioning body, increased memory and more energy. In addition to increasing your indoor oxygen levels, plants can also filter toxins from your environment, such as low levels of chemicals like carbon monoxide and formaldehyde.

Even if you don't have a green thumb, there are plants that are hardy and able to withstand some neglect. So go out and get a house plant, or start growing your own herbs indoors. You will feel better, breathe better, and concentrate better!

Take Action: Start a garden with edible plants. You don't need a lot of space, or even a yard. Try growing your own herbs in your kitchen window, or plant a tomato plant in a pot outside.

AFFIRMOTION

I take pride in the care I give my plants. I nourish them, and in turn they nourish me.

RELATIONSHIPS

Get Social and Off the Media

Strike a Balance

Just Say No

Choose Friendships Wisely

Get Social and Off the Media

There are hundreds of statistics out there about the negative effects of social media on your health. These negative effects are largely attributed to the isolation caused from using the Internet, and the constant comparing of your life to others you see on social media.

The need to always project a perfect life, as seen on social media, is unrealistic and contributes to stress, anxiety, and depression. She has a new car. He has a four-bedroom house. She got a new job. They travel all the time. Sound familiar?

A study from the University of Michigan states that the more time people spend online, the lonelier and more depressed they feel. Further, Facebook contributes to decreased feelings of well-being and "fear of being left out." Anxiety has been shown to increase by comparing your life to pictures you see on Instagram. A survey by the Today Show of 7,000 mothers, found that 42 percent of them reported occasionally suffering from "Pinterest Stress," or anxiety associated with using Pinterest.

It's hard to learn to celebrate others' accomplishments and good fortune without comparing or feeling jealous. Next time you find yourself being critical of others' success, remind yourself that abundance abounds and that there is enough for everyone. Until you can do this consistently, shy away from the social media and create real connections with people face-to-face. Do it for the good of your health.

Take Action: Your time is valuable. Invest it in activities that enrich your existence. Avoid the temptation of constantly checking social media. Reserve a small amount of time once or twice per day to do your Facebooking, Tweeting, Pintering, etc.

AFFIRMOTION

I am comfortable in my own skin. I easily find people and places to interact with socially that allow the real me to shine.

Strike a Balance

Are you a giver or a taker? In the universe there is a yin and a yang, a push and a pull that is going on at all times. You may be a person who is very generous and gives a lot of yourself to others or you may be a more selfish person that does not. Neither one is good nor bad in a single moment, but striking a balance throughout your life's entirety should be something for which to strive.

Exercise your awareness. Make a small adjustment and see how it feels to you. Givers may need to become open to receiving, and takers may need to start giving more. Balance is key. Learning a more balanced way of being, not only with yourself but also with others, will make for better relationships all around.

Take Action: It has been said that happiness occurs when you give kind gestures to help others be happy. Give a gift to someone that you know could use it. This gift can be as simple as a card, or as large as giving some money. Do it anonymously so you are not feeding into your ego, and the act is then selfless instead of selfish.

<u>AFFIRMOTION</u>

Reciprocity is my divine nature. I receive from the bounty, and give from the overflow of the universe. Life for me is in harmony.

Just Say No

Saying "no" is a learned behavior that can benefit everyone. Always being on the go, answering email, texting, closing a deal, running around with your kids, or whatever your distractions are that keep the cycle of busy going, learn to say "no" sometimes. Strike a healthy balance between overcommitting yourself to busy activities and saying no. It can afford you the break you need, and provide other life opportunities to you that you may have otherwise missed.

Manage your time wisely, say no to time-draining commitments a little more, and be guilt free about it. Try saying, "No. Thank you for asking." next time someone invites you to participate in something that you know you cannot commit to with integrity.

Remember, you cannot take care of others to the best of your ability, if you are not running on all cylinders.

Take Action: Say no to that thing you said you were going to do/attend/participate in that you really do not want to do. You know the one I'm talking about! And learn to listen to your intuition, that voice inside, that told you not to commit to it in the first place.

<u>AFFIRMOTION</u>

I gracefully release anything that does not serve me, and joyfully accept my inner guidance and those choices that are for my highest good.

Choose Friendships Wisely

Surrounding yourself with the right people is important to your overall well-being. Friendships are especially important because friends are a crucial part of your support network, and you are choosing to care about and spend your precious time with these people. Friendships should be mutually beneficial, and you should always be on the lookout for new ones to keep things fresh, and for those who help to elevate you to your highest potential.

Do your friends support you and your goals? Are they uplifting you? Do they have similar interests and passions? We make friends at different times in our lives for different reasons, depending upon our interests and needs at that time. Be mindful of the point when a friendship is no longer working for you, and don't be afraid to let it go. When one friendship ends, we are often presented with several other opportunities for new friendships. And just because a friendship has lasted a long time doesn't mean it is good for you.

Starting a friendship is mutual, but ending one doesn't have to be.

Making new friends plays a significant role in your overall health, especially as you age. Trying new things is the best way to make new friends. Friends are also great enablers of good. Embark on your journey to better health with a friend. You will hold each other accountable, and have some fun along the way!

Take Action: Do a survey and see if you are lifted up or put down by your individual friendships. How are you showing up in this connection? Are you being true to your authentic self? Do you have a friendship that may need to be terminated? Make a conscious choice to do what is best for you.

AFFIRMOTION

I am surrounded by supportive, healthy, and loving individuals. All of my friendships are connected spiritually and for the highest good of myself and my friends.

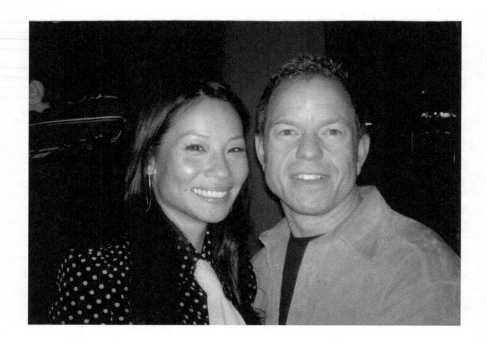

"Teddy Bass has managed to compile 20 years of his unique spirit of motivation into this wonderful book. It's chock-full of simple fitness tips that connect your mind and heart to engage you from the inside-out to help you become the absolute best version of you in your own body. Nothing feels better than that."

- Lucy Lui, Actress, Director and Producer

— 3 —
SPIRIT

"Breathing in, I calm body and mind. Breathing out, I smile. Dwelling in the present moment I know this is the only moment."
— Thich Nhat Hanh

BEGIN WITH YOU

Love Thy Self

Let Go of The Old and In with The
New (Beliefs)

Embrace Your Uniqueness

Face Your Fears

Because You Gotta Have Faith

Play That Funky Music

Love Thy Self

When you look in the mirror, what's your first thought? "I love you." Sadly, this is not the reality for most people. You may see wrinkles, skin blemishes, grey hairs, or something else unappealing to you -- or maybe it is something internal with which you are struggling.

The perceived imperfections and criticisms you have of yourself usually stem from deep emotional holes. Often, people look externally to fill these holes. Sometimes they find comfort in food, relationships, exercise, alcohol, drugs, or activities, but these temporary fixes never last very long. The only way to permanently fill those holes is from the inside of yourself, with forgiveness and unconditional love.

I once did a workshop where the facilitator instructed us to try this exercise in self-love. Look in a mirror and say "I love you" out loud three times every time you pass a mirror. It is harder than it may seem. You just have to do it, and stick with it. You might laugh or look away at first, but keep going.

If you can love yourself unconditionally, then you will not be in constant search of something that will make you feel better, such as, someone else to make you complete, or eating for emotional reasons, or other distractions and/or punishments. Completeness can only come from filling your holes from the inside out.

Take Action: For SEVEN days, every time you see yourself in the mirror, say "I love YOU!" and write yourself a love letter. Seek out mirrors throughout the day! This may sound a little silly, but really pour your heart out. In your letter, tell yourself what you love about yourself, down to the smallest details. Save the letter, and read it to yourself when you need a little pick-me-up.

AFFIRMOTION

I am enough. I can be, do, and have anything my heart desires. The universe is on my side, now and always.

Let Go of The Old and In with The New (Beliefs)

What messages are constantly playing on your internal sound track? Are you stuck inside a certain-way-of-thinking box? Habitual thoughts that you probably picked up from your childhood environment can be destructive and self-restricting, but you have the power to evaluate and change your way of thinking.

As you grew up you were bombarded with the opinions and values of your parents, teachers, role models, friends, and others, which have formed your belief system as an adult. Some of these beliefs serve you in a positive way, while some may be doing the opposite, becoming negative self-talk. The latter can manifest in destructive statements like, "Men are more successful in business than women," or "Rich people have it made," or "I'm not good enough." You have the ability to evaluate your beliefs and get rid of the destructive ones.

Make sure you haven't outgrown old beliefs by being conscious of where your beliefs came from, and if they still serve you in a positive way. Ditch the negative self-talk by releasing all the old baggage and pains from your childhood or unsuccessful relationships, and the beliefs you formed along with them. Take notes or journal, and become mindful of to whom your beliefs actually belong, and then create new beliefs where needed.

Take Action: Get closure. If you can't talk through your hurt with the person associated with the beliefs or emotions that no longer serve you, then write a letter. Say whatever you want to say. Go on a writing rampage! Destroy the letter when you are finished. Remember, the energy that you clear has the power to effect other people, energetically, everywhere!

AFFIRMOTION

I easily find myself journaling. I write and release, burn and forgive, and embrace my true greatness now.

Embrace Your Uniqueness

Have you ever stopped to consider there is not another person on the planet with the same identity as you? You were born this way -- an individual. No other person has your fingerprints in the more than six billion people living today, or in the billions more that have lived or will live. I invite you to fully exist in your individuality at that degree of specialness. You are totally unique in every way, and a necessary part of what makes this world turn.

What stands out to you about yourself that is unique? Is it your nose, height, feet, teeth, or eyes? Do not let the very thing that makes you unique be something you choose to not like about yourself. Embrace that feature, characteristic, charm, or that unique thing that only you possess, in the way that only you can, and realize that you are special and necessary.

I finally learned to love my "annoying" laugh! If I can do it, you can do it too!

Take Action: Pick a feature about yourself that is different from many other people. Examine it in detail. Now, try it on like a new dress or suit, and feel your perfection in this moment.

AFFIRMOTION

I appreciate _____ about myself more every day. I embrace myself completely, and allow self love and confidence to diminish past stories.

Face Your Fears

Do you spend more time living life, or avoiding it? Are you glued to the TV every free moment, watching the latest news or reality television show, vicariously living another life? It is so easy to use technology, or food, or other instantly gratifying activities, to avoid facing fears or problems in our lives. I am telling you right now that you can take responsibility for your own happiness.

We have a tendency to avoid things that may be painful, when right on the other side of that pain is absolute freedom. A wise man once said, "Pain is inevitable, but suffering is optional." Not dealing with issues makes for unhappiness and dysfunctional relationships. Avoidance is a lack of communication, for fear of being hurt or embarrassed. It is important to have your own identity and your own moments. Your life is only as limiting as you allow it to be.

Take Action: Dive into your fears. Be brave and face them head-on! Analyze them. What is the worst that can happen? Really think about it. Accept it. Breathe. Release and let it go.

AFFIRMOTION

I am courageous. I allow all things that come into my life to be stepping stones to wisdom. My growth is inevitable when I let it be so.

Because You Gotta Have Faith

There are many religious sects and beliefs that we have the choice to adopt and practice. Make sure that what you practice is aligned with your soul and your beliefs, and not just an idea you followed and adopted from your parents, your partners, or friends. If you or someone you know has faith in religion, that's great, but be careful of judgment and separatism.

Religious words need not be spoken to discriminate or promote hatred toward others. We are all equal - merely a spec in this vast universe. Adapt the faith you may have been raised with to resonate with yourself now. Your religion should serve you, just as you serve it.

Faith does not have to necessarily be based on a religion. To me, faith is more about conviction in your beliefs that is intentionally practiced. It is knowing what your beliefs are -- having understanding and belief in something rather than nothing.

Some things you don't have power over, but have faith that there is a power acting outside of yourself that allows the best and highest good for you to manifest. Have faith in the unknown. Be observant and patient. Don't always rely on what you see, rather have faith in what you don't see, and be able to connect with something higher than yourself.

Spiritual practice is an investment in your faith. Make a deposit, and you will get interest in return!

Take Action: Explore your spiritual beliefs. Write down the fundamental rules that define your humanity. Ponder the meaning of life and its creation. Begin to form a sacred practice around your beliefs, such as meditation, prayer, or study.

AFFIRMOTION

My trust in a greater power has created faith in myself and my decisions. I accept and allow that my connection to this greater power gives me the awareness that all my needs are met.

Play That Funky Music

What motivates you? Is there something that gets you out of bed in the morning, or gets you to the gym for a workout? Find positive things to help you get and stay motivated. Some of my favorite positive motivators include music, the buddy system, and positive notes.

Music is a huge motivator when exercising for me as well as several of my celebrity clients. I suggest you choose your favorite beats and make a personal workout playlist that speaks to you. Play that jazz or funk, or whatever gets you going.

Having a motivational buddy is hugely effective for keeping you on track with any fitness goal. Whether it is getting to the gym, going on a daily walk, or avoiding the donuts at work, having a friend who has similar goals will keep you both on track.

Use post-it notes for inspiration. Leave messages of encouragement around your home that will be daily motivators like "Appointment with Self at Gym" or "I Will Ride My Bike Today."

Take Action: Replace an unhealthy or negative motivator with a healthy or positive one. For example, if you get to work on time because you are motivated by not getting yelled at by your boss, try instead to be motivated to get there early because you will have first dibs on the best parking spot in the shade. After all, it is only your perspective that you are able to shift.

AFFIRMOTION

I consciously make decisions from the awareness that all of my needs are met, and that I can have, do, and be anything my heart desires, now and always.

END UP FULFILLED

Your Perfect Life

Find Life's Passion

Take Inventory

Creative Vision

Your Perfect Life

It is easy to know what you do not want, but it is so much more important to focus on what you do want. The Law of Attraction suggests that, that which you think of most will form your reality! What do you want your life to look like? Who do you want to attract into your life? What does your ideal home look like? How do you look and feel?

Turn around negative statements in your mind, and make them positive. For example, rather than stating that you do not want to end up with a lemon on your next car purchase, state "I will be drawn to a mechanically immaculate vehicle that perfectly fits within my budget of $250 per month." Your mental garden knows no difference between weeds and prize organic desires. Clearly knowing what you desire, and what your ideal life looks like in the positive, is the first step in making your ideal life a reality.

The second step is writing it down. The written word is powerful. This is how we identify any contradicting thoughts or beliefs with our being, and make it known to the universe that this is truly what we desire.

When you take the time and energy to put what you want on paper, you are sending that energy out into the universe. The universe has a way of bringing you what you ask for in writing. If you can think it (and write it down), you can be and have it, but you have got to "see" it before you can receive it.

A close friend of mine used to say, "Act *as if*, and watch it happen!" You will become a vibration that attracts that which you desire.

Take Action: Write about your perfect life in the present tense, as if you are already living your perfect life right now. Make sure you cover as many areas as possible, such as: finances, business, family, relationships, home, health, love, animals, belongings, travel, etc. Be specific, and be positive. You will soon experience more ease in reaching your goals. Your ideal life is within your control.

AFFIRMOTION

As I spend time thinking and envisioning what I truly desire, I create a high vibration that keeps my mind clear, healthy, and receptive to the good that is always seeking me.

Find Life's Passion

We each have a reason for being, or a drive to fulfill our soul's calling. You can call this your mission, or life purpose. What would you do, or do you do, for free? What would you do if you could not fail? What are you passionate about? What inspires you and brings you joy? What brings you peace and serenity? What would you like to contribute to humanity? The answers to these questions will help you find your life purpose, which reflects the bare essence of what your life is about, and will support the big picture of your life.

Use your life purpose statement to help guide you toward people, places and situations that will make you truly happy. See how decision-making becomes easier and clearer when you know your mission. Don't let fear hinder the process of discovering your soul purpose. There is no dream too big.

Cast aside past failures, judgment, or confusion. Get away from temporary happiness and addictions. The choice to change can be difficult and time-consuming, but it is worth the journey. Have faith in yourself, and the deep knowing within you, to make the right decisions for your life.

Take Action: Create your life purpose statement. To help find your calling, contemplate the questions above. Think about your purpose deeply and honestly. Write down your answers. Refine what you wrote so that it is one sentence, simple, real, and to the point.

AFFIRMOTION

I choose to be happy. I am willing to live, love, laugh, learn, and play more every day.

Take Inventory

Is there a gap between where you are in your life and where you want to be? You may be working in a job where you aren't happy, or in a relationship that doesn't work for you. Take some time for yourself, and discover or uncover what you desire. Do you want to be your own boss? Do you want to attract a partner with a certain list of qualities? Now is the time to figure out the things that make you want jump out of bed in the morning with enthusiasm.

It is okay to not be exactly where you want to be. Be okay with where you are right now, in this moment. After all, life is a journey. But you can't get where you want to be until you know where that is. Take responsibility for where you are in your life, and time to appreciate the experiences that have shaped your life so you can move on. Remember that other people, things, and situations are not the reasons that you have unfulfilled desires.

You can be, have, and do all you desire. You are the steward of your journey and a conscious co-creator of it.

Take Action: Write down your life inventory as it is right now. Examine your life in detail. Compare this inventory to the Life Vision you made about your ideal life. Are there gaps that need to be filled to get you where you want to be? Identify these gaps so you can start to be open to opportunities that will bridge those gaps. It is going to be easier than you think!

AFFIRMOTION

I step into the flow of divine energy that carries my life seamlessly, from where I am to all that I desire, in true fulfillment.

Creative Vision

Finding a creative outlet that inspires you is important. Creativity comes from having a passion, and is a great tool to bridge dissatisfaction with happiness and worthiness. If you are one of those people who doesn't know what you are passionate about, then think back to when you did something and thought "wow, that was fun."

A vision board is a great way to express your creativity, and also help manifest an idea in some area of your life. Your vision board can be a living, breathing, masterpiece that you add to and change as you like, or you can make multiple vision boards for different areas of your life. There are no rules here! Make sure that when you are finished with your collage creation, you put it in a place that you see frequently throughout the day. Then sit back, relax, and let your subconscious and the universe make your ideal life a reality!

Take Action: Create your vision board. Focus on what you want your life to look like, then flip through some old magazines and cut out images that speak to your essence. When you're feeling inspired, paste your images on pasteboard, or tack them to a cork board. Once you have finished, place your vision board somewhere you will see it every day.

AFFIRMOTION

I clearly know my true self, and openly accept the gifts the universe brings me. Within me lies the ability to be a magnetic match for all that I desire. I easily take action on what I am yearning to fulfill and desire to release.

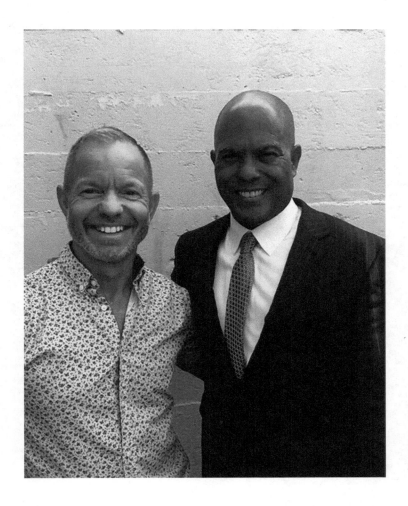

"This superbly written book includes all that is worth knowing and practicing for achieving a healthy balance in body, mind, and spirit. Liberally spread with "affirmotions" for grounding its Take Action exercises, Teddy Bass and Amika Ryan absolutely deliver on the promises made in Affirmed Fitness. Read it, practice it, and thrive."

- Michael Bernard Beckwith
Founder, Agape International Spiritual Center
Author of Spiritual Liberation and Life Visioning

— 4 —
BONUS CHAPTER

---

*"We cannot do everything at once,
but we can do something at once."*
— Calvin Coolidge

LIFESTYLE TIPS

The Organic List to Live By

A Little Burn Here, A Little Burn There

Ditch the Fast Food

Everyday Ergonomics

Pet Talk

A Recipe for Less Toxins

Let Your Life Experience Serve You

Indulge in Moderation

Smaller Footprints

The Organic List to Live By

Certain types of organic produce can reduce the amount of toxins you consume on a daily basis by as much as 80 percent, according to the Environmental Working Group. This ultimately reduces your risk of cancer and other diseases. That's enough to make me want to remember what fruits and vegetables are safe to consume non-organic and which I absolutely have to have organic.

I totally understand that you may be on a budget, and may need to make your hard-earned money stretch as far as possible. So to help you use your shopping budget wisely, I've used data from the U.S. Department of Agriculture on the amount of pesticide residue found in non-organic fruits and vegetables after they have been washed, to make a list for you to live by.

Organic Is A Must:

Cherries, Peaches, Strawberries, Apples, Blueberries (domestic), Nectarines, Grapes (imported), Spinach, Kale, Collard Greens, Lettuce, Celery, Potatoes, Bell Peppers

Non-Organic Usually OK:

Avocados, Pineapples, Mangos, Kiwis, Grapefruit, Watermelon, Cantaloupe, Onions, Cabbage, Asparagus, Eggplant, Sweet Corn, Sweet Potatoes, Sweet Peas

Non-Organic Usually OK:

It's always a good idea to wash your produce before eating it!

Take Action: Write down or print out these two lists, and take them with you for reference on your next shopping excursion. Make sure you are going organic when it counts the most.

AFFIRMOTION

I easily find myself purchasing and consuming fruits and vegetables that are free from toxins, and are nutrient-dense.

A Little Burn Here, A Little Burn There

"Move it and lose it," as I always say. Weight gain is often a result of too much food and a sedentary lifestyle. If you move more, you will see the results you want. Calories can be burned everywhere. Simple minor changes to your day-to-day errands produce major benefits.

Take Action: You can burn calories by adding a little extra effort to daily activities: return that shopping cart; take the stairs; park at the back of the lot.

AFFIRMOTION

I am active daily, enhancing my healthy body, mind, and integrated spirit. This sets an example for the life I desire to live. I am fit and fabulous.

Ditch the Fast Food

The only way "super-sized" should be in your vocabulary is when you are talking about monster trucks. Fast food junkies love those prices and large portion sizes, but all they are getting is lots of calories, sugar, and sodium, along with very little nutritional value. Have you ever wondered why there are no nutritional labels on the bags of food handed out at the drive-thru window?

Nothing that comes from a fast food restaurant is something that you want in your body. Even the fast food places that claim to have "all-natural" products should be avoided. Food nourishes your body. You want it to be clean, organic, fresh, and prepared with love and kindness. Do any of those words remind you of fast food? I hope not!

Skip the drive-thru and plan a few extra minutes each day to prepare healthy meals and snacks with intention, self-love, and worthiness. You deserve it! You will feel so much better when your body doesn't have to process all of those chemical preservatives, unhealthy fats, sugars, and nutrient-deficient starches found in fast food. You are worth the extra time and effort.

Take Action: Plan your meals. Having a meal plan will help you with grocery shopping, reduce food waste, and ensure you always have a healthy, homemade snack on hand. Plan out your three meals and two snacks a day for this week. Write them down, go shopping, and stick to it as best you can. Notice if you feel better, if you saved money, and if you feel more satisfied.

AFFIRMOTION

I enjoy shopping for and preparing fresh, nutrient-dense and organic foods. My body is active, and thrives from the inside out.

Everyday Ergonomics

Your health can be influenced by how you sit at your desk, your sleeping position, and even how you get in and out of your car. Any movements you do repetitively or spend a lot of time in, when done without regard to ergonomics, can be detrimental to your ligaments and tendons, cause pain, and even lead to arthritis. To prevent this, you will need to make sure you are performing movements with good form, and that your posture is correct when sitting or sleeping.

Simply being educated about what good posture is, and mindful of your own posture throughout the day, can make a world of difference reducing stress and strain on your spine. Ergonomic sitting and standing habits will allow you to work more efficiently with less fatigue because this lessens the strain on your ligaments and muscles. In general, a neutral position should be maintained when sitting, standing or lying for long periods of time. You can visualize 'neutral' posture by seeing a straight line from your ear to your shoulder, hip, and ankle. This line should be perfectly perpendicular if standing, or parallel to the ground if lying down. Use this as a guideline to start, as it is also prudent to make sure you are comfortable.

Good ergonomics when seated at your work desk might include you using a stability ball for a chair, or investing in a desk that has height adjustment to allow you either sit or stand to work. You should also make sure your computer screen is at eye level, so that you are not looking up or down and that your chair is adjusted for your feet to rest flat on the floor. When your hands are on your desk, your forearms should be no higher than parallel to the desk surface. Roll your shoulders back and down and be sure your aren't slouching through your upper or lower back.

Take Action: Yoga is a good practice that addresses both the flexibility and strength needed to maintain good posture. Practice simple stretches throughout the work day at your desk, sitting, and standing.

AFFIRMOTION

I am kind to my body. My body knows the best way to move. I listen to and honor my body's signals to me.

Pet Talk

Owning a pet, such as a cat or dog, can greatly benefit your health. The right pet can help you and your family be more active, social, responsible, relaxed, and kind.

No matter your present living and family situation, there is probably a type of pet out there that will benefit you. Empty nesters will find that caring for a pet, such as a cat or dog, fills a void that kids, who are now grown and out of the house, once occupied. If you are single and not home much, maybe a fish or a more low-maintenance pet would be a good fit. Watching a fish swim can be very meditative. If you have kids and have a busy home, the right temperament dog could be a great in aiding your children's learning of responsibility and kindness. A new pet is a great social ice-breaker for seniors. Seniors may find that a sweet dog will provide them companionship and help them to be more social.

Carefully consider your schedule, living environment, finances, and preferences before deciding on a pet. If you do decide that now is a great time to be a pet owner, please adopt a pet from your local animal shelter.

Take Action: Take a field trip to your local shelter and meet some of the great pets that are available for adoption. Talk to the employees about the type of pet you may be looking for so that they can help you find an animal that may be a good match. Even if you're not looking to adopt a pet right now, volunteering at your local shelter can increase your health and sense of well-being.

AFFIRMOTION

My heart overflows with feelings of love and warmth for all living things.

A Recipe for Less Toxins

Having a child has really made me aware of toxins in everyday home and beauty products. As a parent, I can control a lot of the potential toxins in which my son comes into contact. You better believe that there are very few in my household.

Even though you are already aware of the importance of the purity of what you are putting in and on your body, you may still be hesitant to get rid of all your toxic beauty and home care products. So, here is an idea that will save you some money -- do-it-yourself home essentials. There are many great, non-toxic DIY recipes out there. Below are some of my favorites and why!

Coconut Oil Lotion and Facial Cleanser

Coconut oil makes a great body lotion. It can also be used as a facial cleanser with the addition of an essential oil and castor or jojoba oil. Organic and unrefined is best. Are you hesitant to try it on your skin? Don't be. Coconut oil is antibacterial and antifungal loaded with antioxidants, super moisturizing and works on all skin types.

Castile and Baking Soda Tub Scrub

This mix is great for bathtubs, sinks, and counter tops. Mix to a consistency of creamy frosting: one cup baking soda, 1/4 cup castile soap, a splash of lemon juice or vinegar, and a few drops of an essential oil of your choice. Depending on the area of the house, I like citrus, lavender, tea tree, or peppermint essential oil. This recipe is great because there are zero toxins, which means it is safe to use around pets and kids. Baking soda is the ultimate cleanser, and castile soap is a vegetable-based soap that is eco-friendly and gentle.

Fruit and Vegetable Wash

If you're not buying organic fruit and vegetables, it is especially important to get rid of as many pesticides as possible. The best way is with a fruit and veggie wash. Let your fruits or veggies marinade in the wash for five to ten minutes. This will give the wash time to break down any chemicals on the skins. In addition to getting off the pesticides you will remove bad bacteria, germs, and different types of pathogens that can be lurking on your produce. Here is the easy recipe: one part of water, one part white distilled vinegar, a pinch of baking soda (caution, it fizzes), and several drops grapefruit seed extract. Rinse and enjoy.

Take Action: List the things you use regularly that have toxins in them. Find a toxin-free replacement product today or make a your own.

<u>AFFIRMOTION</u>

My body feels light and healthy. I am aware of what I put in and on my body, and I choose products that are clean and toxin-free.

Let Your Life Experience Serve You

This may seem like a no-brainer, but it is amazing how many adults ignore safety recommendations, safety laws, and even their own experiences. For some of us, old habits are sometimes hard to break. Use your head and think "safety first," or ask yourself, "Am I repeating unsafe behaviors?"

When I get into my car these days, if the dinging of the bell was not enough to remind me, my son also says "I agree with the car, papa!" Obviously, you need to wear your seatbelt when driving. It's the law, and has been proven to save lives. But maybe you don't think you need to wear a helmet. It is better to be safe than sorry. Always wear a helmet when doing anything that could allow you to fall and injure your head at a speed greater than a light jog, such as biking, skiing, skating, and horseback riding.

Adhering to common-sense safety practices helps to prolong life, improve quality of life, and prevent injuries. We all desire to take risks from time to time, but there are risks that aren't worth the price you may pay -- whether it's a ticket, an injury, your life, or the life of another. Most importantly, remember that you are setting an example, good or otherwise, for those who might idolize you, like your kids.

Take Action: Create a family emergency plan. You can find tools to help your family make an emergency plan at ready. gov/make-a-plan. Post important phone numbers, like poison control, local law enforcement, and emergency contact, along with your address, in a common area such as on a refrigerator, or by the phone.

AFFIRMOTION

I create a more peaceful life for myself and all those closest to me by having a solution-centered mentality. I am awake, aware, and alive.

Indulge in Moderation

Balance is key to a sustainable healthy life. Some things that are considered to be bad for you, or unhealthy, can actually be good for you in moderation. I am a strong advocate of moderation since nobody is perfect, and life is short. I like the 80:20 rule, which suggests that you should make healthy decisions 80 percent of the time, and you can indulge 20 percent of the time.

Use good common sense and self-control. For example, don't eat the entire cheesecake. A slice will do. Be careful because some unhealthy treats, like sugar, are addictive - and it's hard to stop once you start. For example, if you are eating a sugary snack, you can count on your blood sugar getting out of whack. You will feel tired and sluggish, and crave more sugar. If you need a bit of help you can pre-measure servings of your favorite sweet-treat so you don't go hog-wild, or make a healthy swap.

Your 20 percent fun indulgences are not going to derail your overall health program. It might even give you a little endorphin boost, help you relax, or put you in a better mood. This actually is contributing to your health, not hurting it. As long as you are enjoying your indulgence and you don't go overboard, then go for it!

Take Action: Take one day this week to be indulgent, while maintaining your normal ultra-healthy habits for the other six days of the week. Notice if this was satisfying for you. If not, try being moderately healthy by adding a small indulgence every day, and see if that is more satisfying for you.

AFFIRMOTION

I joyfully allow moderation to guide my choices, and know that I am fully satisfied. Even my thoughts fully satisfy me.

Smaller Footprints

I'm sure you have heard about your carbon footprint and its effect on greenhouse gasses and global warming. Did you know that you can help save the planet while simultaneously helping yourself live a healthier life, by reducing your carbon footprint? There are many ways to reduce the amount of waste and toxic chemicals you personally contribute to the environment. Some of my favorites also boost your health and wellness.

The first one is one you have probably already heard a thousand times -- walk or bike to work instead of driving your car. It's a no-brainer. If you are walking or biking to work, the store, or grandma's house, you are eliminating the carbon emissions from your vehicle. You are also getting a great workout that will burn calories, tone muscles, and boost your mood.

Next, use toxin-free cleaning and personal care products. Keep your health on track while simultaneously preventing those would-be toxins from ending up in soil, water, or the ocean. Eliminating toxic products from your home that contain parabens, phthalates (fragrance), and chlorine, along with a long list of other toxins, will help you steer clear of related cancers, respiratory issues, or hormone problems. If you want bonus points, make your own cleaning and beauty products, and store them in reused bottles and containers. You can find lots of money- and earth-friendly recipes online.

Grow your own foods and buy local produce. This reduces carbon emissions from trucks, trains, ships, and planes that might be bringing in your food from far-away places. Buying local will also help the economy in your community and help you feel more connected to your neighbors. Eating your own fruits, veggies, and meats that you've grown will bring you satisfaction on a job well done, and help you to appreciate how much work and care goes into producing delicious fresh foods. This is also the perfect way to ensure you are eating a variety of fresh, seasonal, foods, which is great for your overall health.

Lastly, reuse or repurpose items. This will help the planet, and keep your finances looking good at the same time. Why buy new when you already have what you need laying around taking up space and collecting dust? You can get really creative, thinking of ways to make trash into treasures. For example, you can use the empty cardboard toilet paper roll to keep things in order. Just cut the roll up the middle and place around the a roll wrapping paper or unruly electronics cords. And don't be afraid to think big. A ladder turned sideways and hung on a wall can make a great bookshelf.

The bottom line is, what's good for the environment is good for you too. So, think outside the box to reduce your carbon footprint and boost your health.

Take Action: What's in your garage or yard that you can repurpose into something great? Do you have old kitchen pots, bowls, or colanders? If yes, now is the time to make them into funky flower or herb pots.

AFFIRMOTION

I easily find ways to recycle, reuse, and repurpose the things that I already have. I feel great when I can de-clutter my space, make something useful, and help the environment.

50+ TIPS

I've included the following helpful tips for all of you readers approaching or already in your 50s. I'm almost 52 years old, and I'll be the first to admit that changes need to be made in your daily life, for a healthier life, when you're my age!

For example, it becomes more difficult to absorb and digest proteins and minerals as you age, which can lead to fatigue, osteoporosis, and other chronic illness, so a supplement or diet change may be in order. Or maybe now that you're older, you've put on some pounds and can no longer eat the foods that you used to (or as much as you used to), and a change-up in your activity type and level is just what you need.

So, for all you 50-somethings reading this, take extra wonderful care of yourself. You're worth it, and you deserve it.

T-Up for Better Bones

Eye Am A Priority

Hearing Your Love Ones

Stay Sharp As A Tack

Save for Your Future

(50+) T-Up for Better Bones

The Centers for Disease Control (CDC) reports over 300,000 people per year are treated for osteoporosis-related fractures in the United States. You are at increased risk of developing osteoporosis if you are Asian or Caucasian, petite and thin, have a family history of osteoporosis, smoke, drink alcohol, or are on certain medications. Women over 50 are four times more likely to develop osteoporosis than men over 50. In addition to not smoking or drinking, there are lifestyle changes you can make to prevent and even reverse osteopenia (pre-osteoporosis).

Exercise is a crucial part of healthy bone management. Don't be afraid to lift. Exercise prevents bone loss and increases bone density, which prevents bone fractures by stimulating cells to make new bone. It also strengthens your muscles and reduces the risk of falling, which is the number one cause of hip fractures.

Supplements including magnesium, calcium, and vitamin D are essential to your bone health. Calcium and magnesium work together to stimulate a hormone for the bone to absorb calcium and vitamin D plays the role of the transporter in the process. Supplementing with 400 milligrams of magnesium citrate is adequate for most people in order to prevent osteoporosis. Your calcium intake needs to increase by 20 percent after age 50, to around 1200 milligrams.

You can help your bone health through your diet by eating dark leafy greens, like kale and collard greens, kelp and nori, which provide high amounts of both magnesium and calcium. The most concentrated sources of natural vitamin D are found in fatty fishes like tuna, herring, mackerel, salmon, sardines, and anchovies, as well as egg yolks.

Take Action: Keep your body moving, exercise, and know your T-score. A T-score represents the overall strength of your bones. It is determined by a low-radiation X-ray called the DEXA Bone Density Test. If you have broken a bone after age 50, then it is time to talk to your doctor about your T-score.

AFFIRMOTION

I freely take control of my own health. I am proactive, exercising daily, and participating in modalities to ensure great bone strength.

(50+) Eye Am a Priority

Eye health is often ignored unless our sight is affected. But healthy eyes are vital to your quality of life, especially as you age.

As we get older our sight can become impaired, and we may need glasses to help us see clearly. I am the perfect example of what not to do. After years of squinting, headaches, and unread articles, I decided to get a long overdue eye exam. Turns out that I am not only near-sighted, but also have astigmatism that decreased my far-sighted vision as well. My options were contacts and/or glasses. Yes, 51 and wearing glasses, and seeing more than ever!

Make the best of the time you have here and really love and take care of yourself, including your eyes. It's time to drop the excuses and complaining. Get over the embarrassment of needing to wear glasses. You owe it to yourself and the ones you love to be the happiest, healthiest, and fittest version of yourself possible. And hey, glasses are in right now anyway!

Take Action: Take a proactive stance about your eye health by getting an annual eye exam, protecting your eyes from the sun, regularly eating foods rich in lutein, such as spinach and kale, exercising, and eating right to combat diabetes, which can cause cataracts, glaucoma, and retinopathy.

<u>AFFIRMOTION</u>

My eyes are healthy and clear. I take care of them, and they allow me the gift of perfect sight.

(50+) Hearing Your Loved Ones

Hearing loss is a serious issue for those of us who are 50-something. It's not just an issue of having to ask people to speak up or missing parts of conversations because you can't hear well. Hearing experts say that by not recognizing the need for, and wearing hearing aids, leads to thinking and memory problems, depression, and dementia.

Thirty percent of adults in their 50's have hearing loss to the extent that they should be wearing hearing aids. Needing to wear hearing aids is nothing to be embarrassed about. Trying to hide your hearing loss is much more obvious to people than wearing hearing aids. Modern hearing aids have directional microphone technology and the ability to act as a bluetooth and link up with your cell phone, which will leave you feeling more like someone with a superpower than someone who is hearing impaired. Remember that sometimes even mild hearing loss needs to be corrected with hearing aids, especially if your occupation relies on the ability to carefully and accurately listen to other people.

Hearing loss can happen in an instant, or gradually over time. Educate yourself on how to prevent hearing loss, and follow through by wearing ear protection or by avoiding potential hazards. Avoid continual exposure to loud noises (85 to 100 decibels) such as motorcycles, jackhammers, snowmobiles, and other machinery, and wear ear protection around very loud noises (110-140 decibels) such as firearms, power tools, ambulance sirens, firecrackers, music concerts, and jet engines. Taking antibiotics, such as gentamicin, can also cause permanent hearing loss.

Don't wait to get a hearing test if you have hearing loss, or suspect that you may. You could be missing out on special moments and conversations with your spouse, kids, grandkids, or friends. Take charge of your hearing health and make the most of your family time.

A few months ago, I suddenly had a constant ringing in my ear, called *tinnitus*. Thankfully, meditation, acupuncture, and having white noise has allowed me to put mind over matter so that I am not bothered by it anymore.

Take Action: Hearing loss can be kept from getting worse with early detection. Get an annual hearing test and track your hearing from year-to-year.

AFFIRMOTION

I am aware of all the sounds around me.
My body's divine knowledge will tell me
when a sound is too loud,
and I will listen.

(50+) Stay Sharp as a Tack

Continually learning new things will empower you to be confident in a variety of situations, but did you know that mental decline is a normal part of getting older? Want to stay mentally sharp as you age? The brain's volume gradually decreases, and nerve cells in your brain can shrink or lose connection altogether as you age. The good news is that there are a number things you can do to prevent or slow down mental decline.

Good overall health and lifestyle habits correlate with better cognitive functions, specifically, maintaining a healthy weight, eating healthy, and staying active. Stabilized blood sugar and normal cholesterol levels have also been proven to keep you sharp. Regular exercise also helps protect and enhance memory, concentration, and mental sharpness because you are increasing blood flow to the brain and using more brain cells as you exercise. Stay mentally active by trying new things, picking up a new hobby, playing challenging games, and increasing your level of social interaction.

When it comes to your brain cells, use them or lose them! Mental stimulation throughout your lifetime is important to brain health.

Take Action: Is there something new you have wanted to try but haven't gotten around to it yet? Sign up for that woodworking class, take that paddleboard lesson, or join your local book club. You'll make new friends, learn new things, and keep your brain in tip-top shape. Just do it!

AFFIRMOTION

I am the perfect age, receptive to new adventures, and my interest is peaking in activities that empower me now.

(50+) Save for Your Future

Let's face it, spending is fun, but doing so wisely today makes for more money tomorrow. If you are like me, you have to work to provide for the lifestyle that you want. I am lucky enough to have found something that I love to do. However, I cannot imagine still working when I'm 70 or 80 years old. I have a financial plan in place in order to ensure I have a stable financial future.

There are many formulas and expert advice out there, but you have to make financial choices based on what works for you. I try my best to allocate at least 20 percent of my income monthly toward either my child's funds, or paying off an unexpected bill. Whatever is left over goes into my savings. That is just what works for me right now.

Map out your savings plan now. Not only because you will have more time to prepare and save if you start now, but you are also probably more able-minded to make sound financial decisions than you would be in your 70's and 80's. Stanford University found that cognitive ability peeks at age 52. Use those smarts in your 50's to have the rest of your years planned out, so you do not have to make tough decisions later.

The bottom line is, do what's right for your situation, and do not neglect to plan for savings and retirement.

Take Action: Refine your retirement plan. Start or increase contributions to your IRA. Think of your IRA payment like you would any other monthly bill. Use a retirement calculator online to evaluate the retirement savings that you need in have place.

AFFIRMOTION

I am able and willing to plan and stick to my budget. I set aside money monthly that will grow my savings, and make conscious choices to build my prosperity.

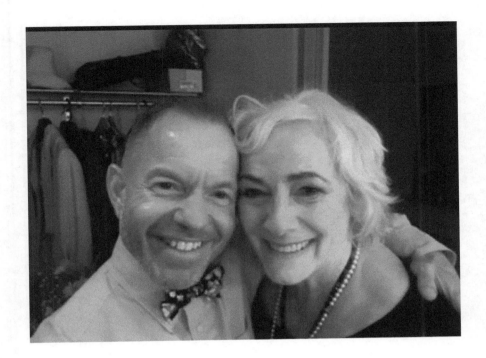

"I love working with Teddy Bass! He is a great trainer, and such an uplifting person. Just being in his presence generates confidence and conviction that you can get the job done. So excited about his new book! Thanks, Teddy, for these years of your loving support, training and tools of spirit that help me do better the work that I do."

- Betty Buckley, Actress, Singer and Storyteller

— 5 —
AFFIR-
MOTIONS

Here are your Affirmotions™ in a list for easy reference. Align your body, mind, and spirit by using your voice, say these Affirmotions™ out load. Use the power of your pen, write them down. Feel these words with every cell of your being. Know them, practice them, and trust the wisdom within yourself for a fitter more whole+sum you!

Today, I choose to be present while eating, bringing my awareness to each meal. I make conscious choices for foods that support my efforts to be fit and healthy, moment-to-moment.

I choose to fuel this vessel of mine with nutrient-dense foods so that my mind and body get a great start each morning. I'm propelled into my day with clarity, vitality, and vigor!

I take the time to shop for fresh produce and prepare healthy and nutritious meals for myself and my family. I allow the food I eat to fuel my creative desire to live this life to my fullest potential.

I easily find myself preparing healthy snacks that provide me with energy, empower me, and contribute to my longevity. I am productive, energized, and at my peak throughout the day.

I easily find myself selecting healthier and more satisfying foods that fully nourish my body, support my mind, and sustain my energy level throughout the day.

I choose to drink water optimized for my best health and which promotes my best self. My body receives the balance of minerals it needs to be hydrated throughout the day.

I am full of energy and enthusiasm, I naturally have an excess of stamina to make every day a great day.

I receive the benefits the universe has for me from the sun and vitamin D. The benefits are here for me to accept and enjoy, and I do so gratefully.

I make proactive health choices that are right for my body. I set myself up for optimal performance, and safeguard my future health.

I easily allow movement to happen in all areas of my life. My body operates at a high level of efficiency and grace, digesting and releasing effortlessly.

• •

I am informed and involved in maintaining my best option in healthcare coverage for myself and my family. I make wise decisions concerning my health, wealth, and well being.

I make daily choices to keep myself moving, grooving, giving, and laughing. I consider all aspects of my life when supporting my heart to beat strong and be vibrant.

I have healthy and beautiful feet. I am grateful that they carry me steadily through all of my adventures in this life.

Good oral hygiene is a priority in my life. I honor myself by flossing and brushing thoroughly at least twice daily.

I show myself great respect through excellent hygiene habits, and these habits benefit my overall well being.

• •

I easily find myself doing thirty minutes of cardiovascular or strength building exercise each day, enhancing my physical and mental well-being. I am committed to living a long, prosperous, and healthful life.

I easily accept the bounty of love, light, and energy that nature has to give me. I let it flow through my entire being as I actively participate in my life.

I easily incorporate more breathing, flexibility, and stretching into my day. I embrace calm and relaxation everywhere at anytime.

I am in tune with my body. I make choices that support my physical and emotional well-being. I create harmony and vigor.

I incorporate multi-joint exercises into my routine that allow my body to stay strong. I perform everyday, functional motions with awareness, comfort, and ease.

My core is strong and resilient. I am conscious of these muscles and their unwavering support, and continue to incorporate core strengthening exercises into my health routine.

• •

I allow myself time to rest, relax, and connect with my body. I am more productive in my daily activities, and embrace a more relaxed and peaceful self.

I am a person who easily presses pause to center my mind, allowing myself to be more present and responsive in my daily life.

I am a desirable being. I choose and desire healthy and positive connections.

I easily take a few moments to remove products that no longer serve me, and select those that are safest and healthiest for myself, my family, and my environment.

As an active participant in my life, I create time for relaxation and rejuvenation. I am refreshed and present in my own life.

I accept the importance of sleep in my life. Its natural benefits restore my body and renew my mind. I fall asleep with ease.

• •

This day I start with a breath. I meditate and allow the day to expand. I realize there is enough time and energy to do all the things that I have listed, with ease and grace.

My life is a constant upward spiral. I set goals that are attainable, realistic, tangible, timely, and rewarding to accomplish.

I am open to attract and receive professionals to help me in any area of my life that needs attention or support. Surrendering to assistance is empowering for me.

• •

I integrate with my youthful spirit, celebrate my choice to live a light-hearted existence, and think positive thoughts often.

Moment by moment, I am more aware of the thoughts that serve me and my highest good. I release all thoughts that limit me or keep me small.

With each breath, I easily connect to my inner calm and peaceful being, and respond in situations to everyone's highest good.

My attitude of gratitude opens doors for opportunities to flow into my life, and inspires me in all that I do.

I easily allow my inner child to laugh out loud and feel the joy from within myself.

I take pride in the care I give my plants. I nourish them, and in turn they nourish me.

• •

I am comfortable in my own skin. I easily find people and places to interact with socially that allow the real me to shine.

Reciprocity is my divine nature. I receive from the bounty, and give from the overflow of the universe. Life for me is in harmony.

I gracefully release anything that does not serve me, and joyfully accept my inner guidance and those choices that are for my highest good.

I am surrounded by supportive, healthy, and loving individuals. All of my friendships are connected spiritually and for the highest good of myself and my friends.

• •

I am enough. I can be, do, and have anything my heart desires. The universe is on my side, now and always.

I easily find myself journaling. I write and release, burn and forgive, and embrace my true greatness now.

I appreciate _____ about myself more every day. I embrace myself completely, and allow self love and confidence to diminish past stories.

I am courageous. I allow all things that come into my life to be stepping stones to wisdom. My growth is inevitable when I let it be so.

My trust in a greater power has created faith in myself and my decisions. I accept and allow that my connection to this greater power gives me the awareness that all my needs are met.

I consciously make decisions from the awareness that all of my needs are met, and that I can have, do, and be anything my heart desires, now and always.

• •

As I spend time thinking and envisioning what I truly desire, I create a high vibration that keeps my mind clear, healthy, and receptive to the good that is always seeking me.

I choose to be happy. I am willing to live, love, laugh, learn, and play more every day.

I step into the flow of divine energy that carries my life seamlessly, from where I am to all that I desire, in true fulfillment.

I clearly know my true self, and openly accept the gifts the universe brings me. Within me lies the ability to be a magnetic match for all that I desire. I easily take action on what I am yearning to fulfill and desire to release.

• •

I easily find myself purchasing and consuming fruits and vegetables that are free from toxins, and are nutrient-dense.

I am active daily, enhancing my healthy body, mind, and integrated spirit. This sets an example for the life I desire to live. I am fit and fabulous.

I enjoy shopping for and preparing fresh, nutrient-dense and organic foods. My body is active, and thrives from the inside out.

I am kind to my body. My body knows the best way to move. I listen to and honor my body's signals to me.

My heart overflows with feelings of love and warmth for all living things.

My body feels light and healthy. I am aware of what I put in and on my body, and choose products that are clean and toxin-free.

I create a more peaceful life for myself and all those closest to me by having a solution-centered mentality. I am awake, aware, and alive.

I joyfully allow moderation to guide my choices, and know that I am fully satisfied. Even my thoughts fully satisfy me.

I easily find ways to recycle, reuse, and repurpose the things that I already have. I feel great when I can de-clutter my space, make something useful, and help the environment.

I freely take control of my own health. I am proactive, exercising daily, and participating in modalities to ensure great bone strength.

My eyes are healthy and clear. I take care of them, and they allow methe gift of perfect sight.

I am aware of all the sounds around me. My body's divine knowledge will tell me when a sound is too loud, and I will listen.

I am the perfect age, receptive to new adventures, and my interest is peaking in activities that empower me now.

I am able and willing to plan and stick to my budget. I set aside money monthly that will grow my savings, and make conscious choices to build my prosperity.

• •

Get more and learn more about *Affirmotions*™ at

Affirmotions.com

Teddybass.com